BUT DOCTOR, YOU'RE WRONG!

Eileen Radziunas

Published by Real Story Press
Haddam, CT. 06438

LCCN: 99-68942

ISBN: 1-57579-179-x

Printed in the United States of America

PINE HILL PRESS, INC.
Freeman, S. Dak. 57029

Acknowledgments

To my family and friends who lived this nightmare with me, providing unrelenting love and support at a time I needed it most—Though I saw your images as blurry and distorted, and heard your voices echo-like and distant, you were angels to my eyes and ears, beckoning me back from the Never Never Land existence my body inexplicably gravitated toward. Because of each of you, I've recovered health and found the courage to share this story. I love you more than words can say!

With special thanks to the many dedicated medical professionals who more than make up for those that fall short. It is due to you that I continue to have hope. From my medical contacts in our local dinner club, to my daughter Stacey, an R.N., currently studying to be a Nurse Practitioner, to my own personal physicians, I recognize and respect many qualified individuals in this field.

My Life / My Fight

With tear-streaked cheeks, leaving their tell-tale impressions in all-too-familiar trails blazed by their many predecessors, as a result of intolerable pain few, beside myself, acknowledge the validity of, I'm compelled to embark on a fight for my life. To accomplish this, it is imperative that I convince disbelieving medical professionals that my current condition is life-threatening, or, at the very least, has the potential to rob me of my ability to write, think, speak or move. Further complicating this unenviable challenge is the fact that I do not have a medical degree and, using layman's terms, must earn the respect and cooperation of those that do.

"Women have always been taught to die politely.
Women aren't doing that anymore."

— Linda Ellerbee —

Several of my best friends are physicians; ironically, so are some of my worst enemies. This is a story about both.

Contents

Prologue

Losing all control, my shoulders heave up and down, spasmodically, in rhythm to the sobs I swallow silently. From the back seat, in a voice quivering with emotion of its own, comes a pathetic, "Mom, don't. If I knew this song was going to upset you so much I wouldn't have included it".

Our eldest daughter Stacey's unnerved comment refers to a gift-wrapped tape she surprised me with as we left the house this morning. Opening it in our packed-beyond-anything-approaching-reasonable car, my eyes moistened as I read the label, "To mom, with love and thanks for all you've done".

Sitting in the passenger seat directly in front of her during the five hour drive I dreaded—my own insecurity surfacing in the fear that distance and the independence of dorm life will threaten the close relationship we share—I am no longer able to deny that letting go is imminent. Throughout the ride, I discreetly wipe the corners of my eyes to prevent the tears from falling in steady tell-tale tracks. My forefingers are bathed in a continuous bath of salty brine that extends to include the backs of my hands as my tears become more profuse. Periodically, one slips by me, streaking its way down my face leaving me to taste the product of a mother's emotional struggle with separation.

As we drive through the gates at the entrance of the breathtaking upstate New York campus, the lyrics "These are the times to remember, for they will not last forever", put me over the edge. Despite previous efforts toward discretion, the impact of the truth I am not yet ready to accept in that message, inevitable as it is, catches me off-guard.

Ignoring Stacey's half-hearted admonishment, my mind temporarily vacates the car, journeying back seventeen and a half years in time to just minutes before Eddie and I left for the hospital, sour lollipop-stuffed LaMaze bag in hand. Between timing contractions, I sneaked one last peek into the brightly decorated, predominantly yellow, fully-equipped nursery. On impulse, I wound the mobile securely fastened to the crib railing. For what seemed like the hundredth time since Eddie assembled it, I watched, mesmerized, as the little stuffed gingham animals spun, like the swing ride at an amusement park, angled out from the umbrella-shaped dome by centrifical force. If eyes could smile, mine were, in their own special way, sparkling at the lovable sight, while my ears welcomed the catchy "It's a Small World" tune they're so familiar with by then.

Eddie's quiet entrance, undetected except for the tender hand he rested on my shoulder, allowed him to share in my reverie. A sudden wince, contorting my face as the next contraction occurred, transported us both back to reality. "It's time to leave for the hospital—now!", Eddie commanded with unmistakable urgency in an out-of-character, assertive voice—or is that panic I hear? Prepared as he was as a childbirth coach, having attended the pillow-toting classes faithfully with me for the previous six weeks, clearly he had no intention of delivering our baby himself.

My face relaxed its muscles back into its usual appearance as I appreciated the break in contractions. Giving Eddie's hand a reassuring squeeze as we exited the room, without realizing it I spoke the words I heard in my mind, "The next time we enter this room, it will be with our baby". The responsive squeeze from his own hand told me I read his own unspoken thoughts.

Hours later and finally fully dilated, I was given permission to respond to the strongest biological urge I've ever experienced, requiring willpower almost beyond human to resist exercising prematurely—the urge to push. Far stronger than desperately needing to go to the bathroom, with no toilet in sight, I was at the point of not being able to hold back much longer, regardless of spot-staring distractions recommended in class, when my obstetrician gave the go ahead I prayed for. And push I did, with every ounce of strength my by-then exhausted body could muster. Encouraged by Eddie and the medical cheering squad surrounding me in the delivery room, any memory of contraction pain was immediately forgotten with my monitrice's enthusiastic pronouncement, "It's a Stacey!"

It was in speechless disbelief, tears streaming down our proud faces, that we listened to the name we pre-selected in the event we were fortunate enough to have a daughter. Her healthy first cry, which, in my euphoric state sounded faraway, like the distant cry of another laboring woman's child, was recorded for her to hear herself, someday.

Cuddling her across my chest, the warmth of her body blending with the sweat of mine, I looked deeply into the big blue eyes of the adorable little face staring up at me for the very first time—and the bonding process began. As the only girl in a family with five younger brothers, having a daughter was a dream come true, a socially acceptable way for me to continue the nurturing process that began as a child, with the dolls I used to name, dress in pretty outfits and love—only Stacey was real, a daughter to treasure for the rest of my life. I felt like the luckiest woman on the face of the earth!

And treasure her I did. From mom and tot swim classes, to molding, by hand, thirty gingerbread boy and girl cookies, each labeled with the name of one of her nursery school classmates, (in addition to one reserved for her), to room mother, scout leader, school trip chaperone, birthday parties with Mexican pinata themes, rented clowns, hay rides and sleepovers, to going out for breakfast and shopping for prom dresses, to confidential talks into the wee hours, the bonding continued. Yet it seemed like I blinked my eyes and overnight her childhood became nothing more than a moment-in-time blur, with Stacey the little girl transformed into Stacey the young adult—and I, for one, was not ready for it. Nor was I ready to hug her good-bye just hours later—but I knew I had to. Intentionally, I didn't look back.

I just got into the car with Eddie and our youngest daughter, Storey, and went home—in tears.

Stacey called that night and I wrote everyday, about anything and everything, just to keep the lines of communication open. Having procured her mailing address in advance, there was a letter waiting for her on the first day she arrived. I decorated envelopes, sent CARE packages and comics, baked for the entire floor and played mom "long-distance" in any way I knew how. Meanwhile, I was involved in Storey's activities. As a freshman at a private girls' school, I enjoyed attending the field hockey games she played, meeting the friends she brought home from her new school and getting to know their parents. By Thanksgiving, I could finally listen to the words "These are the Times to Remember" without blubbering.

It was no surprise when, at a much later date, Stacey shared that she'd saved every letter I'd sent to her. I remember the wide-eyed, "Really?", followed by a smile of security when I admitted I, too, kept all of hers'. Though others questioned why I wrote to her everyday, on parents' weekend, when I learned how much they really meant to her, I thanked God I did. "Mom, to be honest, I was too busy the first couple of weeks to get homesick. Our college intentionally planned mandatory, get-acquainted ice-breaker activities for ten days, practically nonstop. The accelerated social schedule was meant to discourage the natural inclination to miss home. And it worked, initially. Actually, it wasn't until a few weeks into the semester, when the planned activities died down and the real world of classes and homework began, that I felt tinges of homesickness. It was during these times that I'd retreat to the privacy of my top bunk, secluded like a kid in his tree house, and re-read your letters. Somehow they made me feel more connected—and every time I read them, I just knew I was going to make it."

And make it she did. By the end of her first semester she was the typical, well-adjusted college student, with both of us having come to terms with the separation. If anything, our relationship was stronger and closer than ever. Distance was not the enemy I'd anticipated. We've successfully compensated in bridging the miles between us, by concertedly staying in touch with each others' lives, through frequent communication.

Hearing her familiar, high-pitched, cheerful "Hi" before the third ring has a chance to materialize, I feel excitement pulsate through my veins as I prepare to share the news that generated the call. We just received confirmation that our first choice timeshare-exchange vacation spot, in a beautiful resort area on the Atlantic Ocean, has been approved. We love Hilton Head Island. Unfortunately, so do so many other families. It's no surprise that the resort we requested is in such demand. What's not to like? The swaying, leafy palm trees? The dolphins frolicking close to shore? The beautiful beaches, golf courses and breathtaking sunsets?

The more amenities I read to her from the picturesque brochure, the faster my adrenaline flows. I can hear my normally quiet heart pump loudly, racing faster with each added feature.

Stacey's reciprocal excitement further stimulates mine. Closing my eyes, I can almost feel the warmth off the sun's rays bubbling beads of perspiration on my slowly browning body.

At the same time, I'm apprehensive about her feeling left out. Unable to suppress the seeds of guilt from rearing their ugly heads, I unsuccessfully fight the part of my conscience that cruelly reminds me that this is the first spring vacation our family will be taking without her. Unfortunately, high school and college spring breaks do not coincide. Whether it's excitement, guilt, or a little of both that accelerates my heartbeat further, I really can't say—nor can anyone predict what occurs the minute I get off the phone, least of all me.

chapter one
I Saw the Light

With childhood fascination one never seems to outgrow, but suppresses under the guise of being a mature adult, I stare in awe at the most amazing light show I've ever seen. Clear, bright, continuous lights cascade toward me. As quickly as one reaches the end of it's journey, it disappears like a bubble bursting, only to be replaced by another. Clustered together, beehive fashion, these colorless, multi-faceted globes remind me of the packaging paper I use to keep our daughter, Stacey's, college CARE packages intact, cushioned with clear, air-filled bubbles that pop loudly when deflated. Though I can see through these overlapping pools, my vision is distorted, like I have water, or some type of salve, coating my eyes.

My momentary fascination comes to an abrupt halt, as childhood wonderment is replaced by adult intellect, and the learned fear that goes along with it. Something's wrong! I shouldn't be seeing these lights. Substantiating this is the lack of reaction by those around me, unnerving evidence that no one else sees them. Yet, I have a front row seat, in this audience of one, to a continuous performance, more impressive than the most spectacular fireworks display I've ever seen. Though I estimate it started about fifteen minutes ago, that's probably an exaggeration, given that stressful situations are often perceived as longer than they really are. Disconcertingly, my newly-distorted vision continues as I repeatedly try to focus through the bubbles. While I have no explanation for what initiated this mysterious phenomenon, the longer it persists, the more uneasy I feel. Something tells me I'm going to regret having seen these lights.

Admonishing myself for being so melodramatic, my practical side takes control, replacing momentary paranoia with healthier, thought-provoking logic. This concerted effort to put things in perspective results in a more positive frame of mind. I feel fine. A little overtired, but certainly no more than to be expected. If anything, I'm exhilarated over having successfully completed my first full day of work since the onset of a connective-tissue disease. Granted, it was not as an elementary school teacher, the profession for which I'm certified. Realistically, that would require physical activity and endurance beyond the limitations of this illness, a discovery conceded to only after several unsuccessful attempts which exacerbated my symptoms, leaving me physically depleted. Working as an office temporary offers a sit down job with flexibility, while allowing the opportunity to contribute to our daughters' education—a responsibility crucial to my self-esteem.

Though undeniably challenged, harshly, at various stages of this disability, (which primarily affects the muscles and joints throughout my body), things have improved remarkably since diagnosis twelve years ago. My condition is currently as under control as an unpredictable and incurable disease such as this can be. I've come a long way from that unforgettable summer, ten years ago, when I was unable to walk—and my physicians questioned whether I ever would again. My life is full, active and rewarding. I don't see myself as a patient controlled by lupus; rather a person with many facets to my life, one of which, though certainly not the most significant, happens to be this illness.

Such an attitude did not evolve by coincidence. When a person emerges positively from a long-term crisis situation, it is usually due to a strong support system. My success is directly proportional to the commitment demonstrated by family and friends. Because they refused to give up on me, I didn't give up on myself. Unrelenting in their love and concern, their persistence gave me the courage to overcome my physical obstacles and go on with my life.

Further reflection on the crucial role they played is abruptly interrupted by Eddie's unmistakably concerned voice, urging "Hon, why don't you go lie down for a little while?" Startled out of my trance by his unexpected request, his next statement, "You don't look well to me", uttered in an even more troubled, bordering-on-panic voice, tells me he's been scrutinizing me from across the table. With my grossly distorted vision I'm barely able to detect his image, let alone the direction of his gaze. Through my eyes, his features aren't discernable. I feel like I'm looking at him through a blocked out television channel. If I didn't already know what he looked like, I could never describe him.

Though it is impossible to distinguish the temporary concern lines imbedding their wavy indentations in Eddie's brow, or the worry registered in his eyes, I don't have to see them to know that they're there. After twenty-three years of marriage, my mind can visualize, from memory, the physical signs typically associated with the degree of apprehension I now hear in his voice.

Silently chastising myself for alarming him needlessly, I agree to lie down just to ease his mind. When the waterfall of lights stop as I approach the bed, I'm further convinced that this is overkill. However, I have second thoughts with their return a half hour later, as forceful as ever. Again, they last about fifteen minutes.

As the final session of my unanticipated light show concludes, I elect to remain in bed. The comfort of the mattress, into which my sore muscles mold their temporary impression, is too irresistible to relinquish. With a sigh of relaxation, I reach for the newspaper. Though momentarily taken aback when I'm unable to decipher most of the words, my concern disapates as I rationalize that I'm probably more tired than I realized.

Though I expect to fall right to sleep, I can't. My eyes burn so intensely, they hurt. The pain, generated from inside them, remains constant. I toss and turn for hours before my body finally gives in to the overwhelming fatigue.

When I awaken several hours later, my first awareness is the intense burning that still penetrates both eyes. Panicking from a potential threat so frightening that I can't even admit it to myself yet, I impulsively open them. As I do, I'm confronted with the unnerving realization that my customary blurry vision, when not wearing prescription lenses for nearsightedness, is remarkably intensified. Unable to focus on the wreath hanging on the wall facing our bed, my heart begins to race. Quickly donning my glasses does little to improve the clarity.

Entering the bathroom, I'm momentarily caught off-guard by the murky reflection ominously staring back from the medicine cabinet mirror. Until now, I thought blurry vision was the sole consequence of last night's inexplicable incident. But as I try to compensate for my decrease in visual acuity, by leaning over the sink to get closer to the glass, I'm confronted with a sickening truth that proves I was grossly mistaken. Overcoming my momentary shock, I study an inarguably transformed appearance. My eyes look like a raccoon's, ringed in dark shadows. Tired and muddy, their clear, healthy spark is gone. Lined with uncharacteristic red, spider-like veins, they provide an eerie contrast against my unusually chalky, pasty white complexion.

For the first time since last night's unprecedented light show, I'm overcome by terror. Will my vision ever return to what it was? Will it worsen? Am I losing my sight? With a shudder of fear vibrating through me from head-to-toe, too afraid to even consider these disturbing possibilities any longer, I dial the ophthalmologists office. If ever I needed the expertise of this specialist I've come to trust, impeccably, with my vision, it's now. A sinking feeling materializes in the pit of my stomach as the receptionist informs me that the doctor I've seen for twenty-plus years isn't in today. Silently lamenting the inaccessibility of not only his technical skill, but, the emotional support I can always count on from this physician and friend, frustration gnaws away at me. Making a concerted effort to disguise my intense disappointment, unable to deny my symptoms demand immediate attention, I schedule a late morning appointment with his associate.

Driving the ten minutes to his office, I'm uncharacteristically insecure behind the wheel. Though I can read the road signs, it is only through blurry vision. My depth perception is distorted. An uncomfortable, strained sensation escalates the more I use my eyes, particularly with the visual intensity driving requires. Not only do they ache, they fight me to close. It takes unnatural concentration to resist the strong muscular pull to do so.

Sitting in the ophthalmologists waiting room, I apprehensively conduct my own vision test, staring at various objects to see if I can make them come in clearer. I can't. Even the familiar receptionist, whom I've come to know on a first name basis, looks fuzzy to me. If I didn't know better, I'd swear the glass window she sits behind is really a large aquarium filled with water, distorting her appearance. The high gloss sheen of the magazine pages I mindlessly flip on my lap, make reading impossible. Fortunately, before I can give myself any more anxiety-producing tests, I'm called in.

After the preliminary, ice-breaking introduction customary of first visits, the doctor asks, "What brings you here today?" Struggling to keep my voice steady, I describe the "lights" incident, stressing the alarming residual visual changes. Listening intently, he interrupts only for further clarification.

His lack of any significant abnormal findings, after thoroughly examining both eyes, is reassuring. As the tight knot of anxiety starts to loosen in my stomach, I can almost visualize it untangling. Overcome with relief to hear he suspects I had a migraine, I have all I can do to concentrate on anything else he says. When the follow-up appointment he schedules is in six weeks, I am further convinced he doesn't see this as a serious, or immediate, problem.

Leaving the building I feel strange, almost disoriented—spacey, in a way. To my embarrassment, I stagger out to the parking lot, more like an alcoholic exiting a local bar, than a patient leaving a doctor's office. How ironic, I'm more concerned about camoflauging my aberrant behavior from the few patients around me than dealing with the real issue, i.e. what on earth is happening to me? Talk about being too socially conscious for one's own good! Or is it just plain denial?

The parking lot seems exaggerated in size; the curb is not where it's supposed to be. When I step down, my foot touches the ground before I expect it to, with an awkward stomp that takes me by surprise. I feel like I just got stronger lenses that my eyes haven't adjusted to, yet. Involuntarily leaning to the side, I reach out to steady myself against several parked cars as I insecurely inch my way to mine. Finally, after seriously questioning whether I would, I reach our New Yorker.

Driving intensifies the visual disorientation. As I grip the steering wheel tighter than usual, I feel my confidence waning. By the time I pull into my driveway, and over-cautiously steer the car through the ordinarily ample garage door opening, my nerves are shot. Lying down, I notice another unexplained phenomenon, a tingly, tickle-like sensation in my hands and feet. Inspecting my hands under the bedside table light, as though this superficial topical scrutiny could offer some clue as to why they feel so strange inside, I study palms transformed into a mosaic of blotchy red and white spots.

Observing the small, irregular-shaped specks, I'm convinced I've seen them before. But when? Obsessed with making the connection, I tax my memory banks, driven to the point that I can think of nothing else. My persistence pays off when it dawns on me that they resemble the measles I had as a child, except, unlike that no longer prevalent disease, distribution is limited to my palms. Convinced they're not measles, their sudden manifestation intrigues me, particularly in light of my other symptoms.

Although not one to push the panic button, it's getting increasingly difficult to ignore the frightening and inexplicable changes insidiously overtaking my body. As a matter-of-fact, it's impossible. Even simple, everyday activities, previously taken for granted, are affected. Participation in family interactions that are such a part of my world is limited. Storey's field hockey games are no longer enjoyable to watch because the repetitive movement of turning from side to side, while attempting to follow the ball to the goals, nauseates me. I find myself concertedly suppressing the urge to vomit. Unable to write legibly through my visual distortion, Stacey's college mailbox no longer receives daily contributions from mom. I feel too sick to eat, let alone continue our weekly dinner dates at favorite restaurants—quality time Eddie and I both value and miss.

At the moment, I'm unable to read the fine print on a medical insert which accompanies one of my prescriptions. This has no bearing on the fact that, at age forty-four, I've joined the bifocal generation. I already wear lenses that compensate, effectively, for this aspect of my aging eyes. And, unlike when my eyes were bi-focal deficient, moving an item further away to the end of my fully outstretched arm, an age giveaway commonly exhibited by members of my baby-boomer generation, does nothing to improve the clarity. Lately, any attempt to read leaves my eyes uncharacteristically bloodshot and teary. I disagree with the ophthalmologist. Something definitely happened to my eyes. It happened as a result of seeing those lights—and I intend to find out what.

As the hot, steamy bath water clears my nasal passages with its moist, rising vapors, it enticingly beckons my sore, weary muscles. Appreciatively, I descend into its soothing warmth. Even before submerging as deep as the three-quarter filled tub allows, I can feel myself start to relax after a long, tense day.

As my tightly knotted muscles loosen, I unwind. Minus this distraction, my head clears, allowing my thoughts to formulate into a plan. I need to see my medical doctor. Too many areas of my body are involved to limit investigation to opthamology. First thing in the morning I'll call for an appointment. Content with this decision, I crawl into the inviting coziness between our warm flannel sheets, pull the handmade quilt up to my chest and reach for the newspaper.

In this relaxed state, I momentarily forget about my visual disturbances. Reality quickly hits as I unsuccessfully attempt to read the blurry words, whose letters fade in and out. Rubbing my eyes, blinking furiously and moving the newspaper in various positions are fruitless efforts toward making the print clearer. Frustrated, I drop the newspaper, draw the quilt up around my neck and curl into the fetal position.

Tired as I am, I can't sleep. What were originally tingling sensations in my hands and feet are now painfully sharp, stabbing pins-and-needles. As the prickliness climbs, crawling up my wrists to my forearms, ankles to my calves, and spreads to the back of my neck, getting stronger, deeper and more intense by the minute, these voodoo doll-like pins really hurt.

Fear engulfs me as I recall a woman's magazine article I read several years ago, in which the disabled author described the process of becoming paralyzed. In it, she stated that just prior to this devastating occurrence, she experienced sharp pins-and-needles all over her body. Remembering the article for the first time since I read it, my fear escalates in direct proportion to the increasing intensity of the unexplained stabbing phenomenon. Listening to my husband's rhythmic breathing, as he sleeps peacefully beside me, I witness the transformation of night into day, too scared and preoccupied to remember how tired I actually am. As the sun rises and the birds chirp, I ask myself why I am not as convinced as they, that this is going to be a great day.

Driven by fear, but overcoming the momentary inability to remember my doctor's phone number, my sweaty, shaking fingers nervously punch in the appropriate digits. With my emotions already at their extremes, it takes no more than hearing that he is on vacation for my eyes to fill. Why now, when I need him more than ever? Silently admonishing myself for the self-centered attitude which, fortunately, I had the presence of mind not to share, I agree to see one of his associates.

Driving to the office, I unsuccessfully try to blink out my blurry vision. Like before, I can read all the road signs, wavy though they may appear. The more I concentrate on them, the more my eyes ache. My head feels fuzzy, almost like I've been drinking champagne. I'm dizzy and unsteady behind the wheel. It's a relief to spot the blurry sign to his office complex just ahead.

chapter two
Local Medical Consultation

Unable to deny the potential for a serious situation, it is with considerable trepidation that I enter the doctor's office. Lying on the vinyl padded, paper-lined exam table, the little room takes on an eerie silence, broken only by the rustling of the disposable johnnie as the physician opens it to listen to my heart. While he concentrates, I lose myself in the preoccupation of my worried thoughts, only to be startled back to reality by the doctor's voice. "You must be really scared. Your heart is racing."

Though undeniably concerned, if anything, I should be somewhat relieved, considering the physician did not overreact to the history I gave a few minutes ago. As a matter-of-fact he was very reassuring. So why am I lying here trembling uncontrollably? And what's with this unsteadiness I hear in my voice as I respond to his questions? Why is my mouth so dry while the palms of my hands and my armpits are so moist? Why? Because I'm terrified, that's why! And his well-intentioned efforts to relax me fall on deaf ears.

Not for one minute am I buying that this is going to be a "little" problem as he tries his best to convince me. If he really thought that, he wouldn't be ordering a C.A.T.* scan of the brain in his very next breath, explaining "I just want to be certain we're not dealing with a small tumor." Regardless of how many miniscule adjectives he uses, I hear one thing: brain tumor. And I'm scared!

Fighting the urge to cry, I can hardly look at the receptionist-turned-friend over the years, as she calls to schedule a STAT C.A.T. scan of my brain. I barely hear her ask for my date of birth, much less answer coherently. Instead, thoughts of Eddie and our daughters are all consuming: our indescribable love for each other-the good times we've shared-the plans we dream together for our future. This can't be happening to our perfect world. Please, God, not our family! We all have too much to live for; It wouldn't be the same without one

* CAT or CT scan (Computed Tomography): A procedure using radiation to view the brain. An initial stroke diagnostic technique, (among other uses), it denotes cause and location.

of us. "Stop it!", I scream silently to myself, interrupting premature, out-of-character pessimism.

Sitting in the mauve and gray starkly-decorated waiting room, typical of most clinics in its lack of discretion, it is easy to overhear the reasons other patients are here: bloodwork, finger x-ray, glucose tolerance, and a variety of routine tests. Somehow, mine seems so much more ominous, I find myself envying them. Just the fact that this procedure, which generally takes days to schedule, is today, indicates the unsuccessfully camoflauged immediacy involved.

Fortunately, before I have time to feel any sorrier for myself, a technician wearing a crisp white smock opens an inner door, hesitating before attempting to pronounce the name on the file she holds. Coming to her rescue, I knowingly ask, "Are you looking for Eileen Radziunas?" With an appreciative smile of relief, she answers affirmatively, followed by an apologetic explanation I only half listen to. I have more important things on my mind than whether she can pronounce my name. Following her down the antiseptic smelling, light grey corridor, we enter the room with the scanner. I'm asked to remove the religious medal I've recently begun to wear around my neck. Reluctantly, I do so.

A C.A.T. scan is a painless, somewhat relaxing procedure. With the lights dimmed, as the technician vacates the room, even the cold, hard table isn't enough to prevent me from submitting to the fatigue brought on by my sleepless night. Just as I start to drift off, I hear muffled voices at the foot of my bed, behind what appears to be some type of a partial screen. Unable to sit up to get a better view, due to the testing tunnel my head is in, all I can make out as I tuck my chin to my chest and stare out, over and beyond my body, is what appears to be several people pointing to something. Straining to hear their whispered voices, I can only discern bits and pieces. The one line I hear unmistakably, "It looks like there's liquid in this area; Can you see where I mean?", is immediately followed by the others concurring.

Referencing my age and symptoms, there's no doubt whose scan they're discussing. My curiosity only surpassed by understandable anxiety, it's a letdown to hear the technician inform me that although the test is over, it will take three working days for my physician to receive the results. My mind rants and raves in unspoken impatience. I want to know the outcome—NOW! Yet, in reality, I know technicians are not at liberty to disclose results, and to ask would be an effort in futility. Consequently, my silent tirade, the only outlet for my current frustration, continues to ignite my thoughts as I dutifully stop at the lab to have blood drawn before heading home.

Thank God it's Friday! I can't wait for Eddie to get home from work. Inarguably my best friend, the product of a friendship that started long before we dated, back when I was a sixteen year old in braces, living across the street from him, I can't think of anyone I need more right now. Just for this weekend, I'm grateful that Stacey is away at college and Storey is staying at a friend's house. I need to be alone with him. I'm scared and I crave the comfort only his strong embrace can give—the soothing only his gentle voice can impart—the love for one another only we share.

The excited bark of Paddington, our collie, announces Eddie's arrival. Walking out to the porch, I find him affectionately greeting our dog. Paddington's quality time comes to an abrupt halt the minute Eddie sees me. Oh, God, don't let him give me that hopeful, questioning look, the one that implores me to report some good news, when I can't. The look that says, "I love you so much I'm worried sick over you".

Not one to overreact regarding health issues, probably because we lived through so many together, there is no disguising his current fear. Overnight, his youthful-looking face seems to have aged ten years. There are dark circles under eyes that worry has robbed of their sparkle. I can only guess what this loving man, who has come to depend on me—because together we're a team—is fearing. I want to cradle his head in my arms and tell him I'm okay and that everything will work out, but I can't. Instead, we meet in a silent, knowing embrace that says more than any words ever could.

After recapping the events of the doctor's appointment and C.A.T. scan for Eddie, I'm more tired than hungry, and opt to go to bed. Before doing so, I share the conversation I overheard in the scan room with him. He reacts with mixed feelings. While concerned that the C.A.T. scan may be abnormal, he's optimistic at the same time. Hugging me, I cling to the hope in his barely audible, but comforting words, muffled as they are spoken into the top of my hair, "Hon this could be a good sign. The doctors may have found something treatable. As we speak, they could be coming up with a plan to reverse your symptoms".

Exhausted to the point that even my typically much-anticipated bath was an effort tonight, I quickly dry off and slip into a soft flannel nightgown. For the end of March, it is unseasonably frigid. Nestled in the warmth of our cozy bed, this seemingly ideal setting for a good night's sleep is deceptive.

As if the intense burning, (which makes both eyes feel like they were broiled), and the stabbing, pins-and-needles throughout my body were not enough, suddenly my hands, feet and mouth are going numb. Although I can feel them, there is significantly reduced sensitivity, comparable to the way lips feel after dental work, once the novocaine starts to wear off. My throat feels funny, too. It's hard to swallow. Once again, it takes several hours of tossing and turning tonight for sleep to win, and, at that, only for a few hours.

By 5:00 a.m. it's obvious my night is over. Rather than fight the odds, I decide to take my daily three mile walk, a tradition for the last three years. Using the same indoor track as always, I'm uncharacteristically nauseated as I make the loop. Choosing to ignore it, while hoping it will pass, I continue. Instead, it intensifies. I'm so dizzy I have to stop. My legs feel weak. Even pressing both palms against the wall for balance, I sense I could just fall over. In fact, am I tipping or is that my imagination? I never remember feeling so strange in my entire life. And why aren't things where they should be? The familiar objects in the room look misplaced, like they're further away than where I remember them. Something's wrong with the ceiling. It's different—almost tilted. The unexpected impact of my entire body toppling into the wall further takes me by surprise. I feel like I'm about to vomit but, instead, I'm concertedly suppress the salty taste, high in my throat, which historically precedes throwing up. Reluctantly, I forego my aerobic walking for today, determined to attempt it again tomorrow.

Later in the day, Eddie suggests going for a ride, an idea I adamantly veto because I feel so awful. But he persists, countering "It might make you feel better to get out". Though unconvinced, I don't have the energy to resist further. Reluctantly, I agree.

Five minutes into the ride, it's obvious I've made a mistake. Looking out the window is reminiscent of when I was five years old and so prone to carsickness that my parents had to drop me off on one corner and let me walk to the next. Only then, after being out in the fresh air, could I ride a few more blocks. Needless to say, our family drives took an eternity.

Reading the road signs makes me even sicker. I don't dare talk, for fear of throwing up if I even open my mouth. My head is dizzy in any position, especially when I turn from side to side. Consequently, I stare straight ahead, concentrating on distracting myself with the thought of getting home and to bed as soon as possible.

As we pull into the garage Eddie tenderly reaches over for my hand and, in a serious voice matched only by the solemn expression on his face, says "Hon, I'm very, very worried about you. Though I'd hoped the ride would've gotten your mind off whatever is going on, it's apparent that's impossible. Your intensity and lack of conversation are so out-of-character." I agree with him. "Eddie, as hard as it is for you to understand, I feel like a different person. I see it myself. Ever since the lights' episode, it's like I'm in a bubble, removed, but at the same time conscious of what's going on around me. Though I hear everything being said, and respond somewhat appropriately, there's been a drastic and inexplicable change in me." Silently, I reflect on how I especially notice it at the dinner table, where I feel like I'm in a vacuum, in spite of the continuous efforts he and Storey make to draw me into their animated conversations, as they desperately strive for some semblance of what life was like before. But I resist. In my heart, I know I'm not as much a part of them anymore. There's been a dramatic separation—overnight, I became a stranger to myself and to those who knew and loved the old me.

As I watch my family interact without my input, it scares and saddens me. Will I ever be a part of them again? On the same level as before? Or, is God trying to show me that they will be okay, as they laugh and joke among themselves, at times seemingly oblivious to my lack of interaction? With misty eyes, I mourn the loss of the person I once was, as I pray to God that she'll return—for all our sakes.

Dr. Michaels, my primary care physician, has never been one to overreact. That's all the more reason I read today's undisguised concern as cause to worry. Pursing his lips tightly, slowly shaking his head from side to side as I detail the lights' incident, I find the rhythm of his fingers tapping against my chart nerve-wracking. Looking away as I concentrate on sequentially describing the symptoms generated since the lights' incident, I can almost feel the intensity of his concerned eyes boring through me. I wish I could read his mind. I want to know every diagnostic possibility he considers, including those he might be reluctant to share with me—then again, maybe I don't.

In light of the discussion I overheard at the clinic, I'm surprised my C.A.T. scan results are normal. But Dr. Michaels isn't convinced. My symptoms are too neurological to remain unexplained. To more extensively study the brain, he orders an M.R.I.* scan.

The four days between the office visit and the scheduled scan seem like an eternity. Finally, wearing the comfortable clothes that were recommended, in this case a jogging suit, we stop at the pharmacy for the mild sedative ordered to counteract any claustrophobic affects and head for the hospital.

* M.R.I. (Magnetic Resonance Imaging): A procedure using a large magnetic field to provide sharper and more detailed views of brain injury than CAT scans, particularly for small, deep injuries.

Grateful not to have to contend with the nauseating sensation of the high-ceilinged waiting room for more than a few minutes, my name is called and we enter the inner chambers. With wobbly, jello-like legs, I follow the silent, carpeted footsteps of the male technician, consumed with the ominous prospect that my fate is about to be determined.

Suddenly the entire procedure seems more formidable than I anticipated. Though my congenial escort does his best to put me at ease, the nature of the required questions override his efforts to do so. "No, I've never had brain surgery. (Nor do I want it, for that matter!) I have no metal plates in my head and I never had any metal removed from my eyes."

In response to my growing anxiety as I try to second guess what he'll ask next, my stomach emits a loud, nervous gurgle, adding embarrassment to my current discomfort. Tactfully utilizing the undisguised message, communicated through unavoidable eavesdropping as my anatomy asserted itself, he quickly offers me water for the sedative my physician ordered.

As my husband and I follow him into the attached trailer, housing the mobile M.R.I. unit, my icy cold hands and racing heart provide further anatomical confirmation of my escalating fear.

Even before the loud reverberations of our footsteps on the metal gangplank stop echoing their tinny complaints, my blurry vision struggles to focus on the M.R.I. scanner. Coming in closer range, it appears that attached to a tunnel-like capsule is a narrow, conveyor-like patient mover, no wider than a ladder. Apprehensively, it occurs to me that it is long enough to slide a patient completely into the claustrophobic-looking enclosed chamber.

After relinquishing our credit cards, (the magnetic attraction is strong enough to strip them), watches and my religious medal, Eddie and I enter the tiny galley which houses the scanner. Like the rest of the trailer, the room is cold. As a shiver involuntarily tenses my entire body, I question whether its origin is cold—or just plain fear.

Removing my walking shoes, my hands tremble, making it awkward to untie the laces. Eddie and I insert the required earplugs, designed to partially obliterate the notoriously loud scanner noises. Lying on the narrow table, my arms just fit next to my sides, without falling off the edges. When the attendant straps them in loosely across my abdomen, I feel more secure. Next, my head is anchored to prevent movement from side to side or up and down. The restraints are gentle. Nothing hurts. The test is ready to begin.

Before starting, I request a trial run, a tip I received from other M.R.I. patients. It's psychological. Doing a test run reassures the novice patient, firsthand, how quickly they can be removed from the tunnel.

The technician readily complies. With my eyes open, the test ride begins. Inching head first on my journey down the lit tunnel, I'm uncomfortably conscious of the close proximity of my face to the roof. It's only inches away! By the time I've traveled far enough for my knees to enter the tunnel, I feel uneasy. I can no longer see the light from the room. For the first time in decades, I recall watching cowboy shows as a child in the fifties, on my grandparents' coveted black and white, rounded corner television screen, where the villain often met his demise by being buried alive. This mental analogy, the product of an overactive imagination, threatens claustrophobia just as my trial run ends and I re-enter the real world.

When the technician slides me back in for the actual test, I close my eyes and keep them closed for the duration. Doing so makes me less conscious of how far in I am. It also diminishes my awareness of the tomb-like enclosure. Eddie's warm, reassuring hand on my ankle, throughout the entire forty-five minute procedure, helps me feel in touch with the world. His continued verbal communication, intentionally shouted to be heard above the loud banging of the noisy equipment, relaxes me. Before it seems possible, three-quarters of an hour has passed, the scan is completed, we've claimed our belongings and are on our way home.

Closing my eyes to minimize the nauseating affects of the car ride, I reach over for Eddie's right hand and, as though deriving strength from his touch, I admit my desperation for a meaningful test result. "Eddie, this test has GOT to give us some answers", I assert in a more convincing voice than I feel on the inside. With a gentle squeeze of the hand, he cautions me, "Hopefully that's true, but don't count on it." His skepticism is justified. Over the years, we've learned the hard way that all tests are not conclusive, and that lab and technician errors sometimes result in inaccurate interpretation. Choosing to ignore his warning, I convince myself that symptoms as bizarre as mine are bound to be identified.

I suppose by this time I should know better. The results of the M.R.I. are normal—but you can't prove that by me. I feel awful. I'm so nauseated, I can barely change positions, or look from side to side, without vomiting. It makes me sick to my stomach to attempt to have a conversation while sitting between two people. Eye contact is impossible unless I relocate to sit across from them and, even then, the best I can hope for are the blurry images which now constitute the only way I see things. Riding in cars intensifies the situation because, if there's one thing worse than blurry scenery, it's blurry scenery moving quickly. It makes me feel like I can just lose it.

Overnight, my notoriously ravenous appetite has become nonexistent. The only way I know it's mealtime is if someone reminds me. I've lost my internal hunger trigger. There are no cravings for, or salivation at, the thought of formerly irresistible foods. My stomach never growls from hunger. Though I force myself to eat, I can only get down one or two bites. My clothes are literally falling off of me because of the rapid seven to ten pound a week weight loss.

By the day, more unusual symptoms develop. The latest is the swallowing difficulty I first noticed this weekend, characterized by an uncomfortable choking sensation that keeps me up throughout the night. Lying down intensifies it. On the rare occasions that I do sleep, it is only by sitting straight up against several pillows.

Transient numbness continues to affect all areas of my body, though most consistently my left foot. None of my appendages are exempt, however. It's unnerving to awaken, day after day, afflicted by some new, and even more bizarre symptom. This morning my tongue was numb and heavy. Yesterday my face prickled with stabbing pins-and-needles. At the moment, my body is wracked by waves of chills surging episodically from my abdomen to the tips of my extremities. I shudder to think what physical manifestation tomorrow will bring!

Still unable to touch my eyes, they continue to ache and burn incessantly. And what's this pulsating sensation, like liquid bubbling, that I feel throughout my body? The rippling feeling, though momentary, reminds me of when I was pregnant and felt life for the first time. As I can recall, the sensation was so subtle, it left me questioning if that was what I was really feeling. Nineteen years ago, during this initial in-utero introduction to our baby daughter, the memorable moment resulted in spontaneous tears of joy that only another mother can understand. I can remember exactly where I was and what I was doing when I felt that unforgettable first flutter. But the analogy ends here. I'm not pregnant and I shouldn't be feeling ripples in my abdomen, or anywhere else for that matter. Yet, I am.

Even more unnerving is the involuntary muscle jerking. Without warning, an appendage will jump up a few inches from its resting position, forcefully enough to hurt associated joints. While I lament the physical chaos raging war inside my body, I catch a glimpse of equally affected exterior damage, as my frightening image reflects back at me, from a nearby mirror. I can't believe that's really me! I no longer know the blurry person staring back with unfamiliar dull, bloodshot, dark-circled eyes. Occasionally, her smile is askew, or one eye tears and, of course there's that ever-constant, red blotch attached to the middle of the upper lip on her thinner than normal face. My God, what's wrong with me?

Terror escalates with each new and frightening symptom. Unable to contain my fears a moment longer, I call Dr. Michaels and insist on a neurological consult.

chapter three

Neurological Consult

Consumed with pessimism my mind incompassionately refuses to let me escape, fears that such bizarre symptoms may be the result of irreversible neurological damage surface. By pursuing medical intervention with the immediacy I'm convinced my condition demands, I pray this negative pre-occupation proves unfounded.

Sitting on the edge of the side chair adjacent to her massive oak desk, impersonally stark except for a Physician's Desk Reference and two inch oak, block letters that spell out Dr. Bates, I begin to feel uneasy. Unnerved by the inescapable reality that patients don't go to neurologists for minor ailments, I struggle to emotionally brace myself for the realization that before I leave, I may know more than I'm ready to hear. And I'm scared.

Unfortunately, Dr. Bates' mannerisms do nothing to relax me. Straightforward to the point of making me uncomfortable, her body language is rigid. She never smiles. Rarely does she come up for air, too busy firing questions machine-gun style, while scribbling copious notes, without comment. Some of my responses make her eyes bulge with surprise. Others cause them to slit, skeptically. At times, she shakes her head as if in agreement.

With building anxiety her lack of bedside manner only intensifies, I refer to my cheat sheet of symptoms. There are too many things happening throughout my body to trust to memory, particularly in an unnerving interview environment such as this.

The exam is similar to the one Dr. Michaels conducted. In a darkened room, she studies my eyes with a bright, hand-held light that she clicks periodically, I assume to adjust magnification, as I stare at a pre-designated spot. Moving it from side-to-side and up and down, I'm asked to follow it. With my eyes closed, I'm told to touch my finger to my nose. An instrument emitting high pitches is used to check my hearing.

To further verify that all my senses are acute, she queries if the pins she more-than-lightly pricks into both sides of my body feel equally sharp, which they do. Sticking my tongue out and moving it from side to side, though an informative and necessary neurological exercise, makes me feel no less foolish than when asked to do so the other day. Closing my eyes tightly, and then opening them wide, is a less awkward instruction to follow. After testing my reflexes, which, according to her are "brisk", she verifies limb coordination and strength. The last thing I'm asked to do is to walk on my toes, heels and flat-footed, which is no problem.

As a result of unimpressive clinical findings, she concludes that a migraine headache was responsible for the lights I saw. With conviction, she asserts "Certainly, no serious neurological phenomenon is occurring." Her recommendation, delivered with confidence, is extremely high dose steroid therapy, (80 to 100 mg.), limited to a few days, with the intent of "shocking my system".

She may be convinced but I'm skeptical. "Doctor, my understanding of the visual distortion associated with migraines is that it's transient. I've never heard of a migraine that left a patient's vision permanently blurry. Besides, I'm already on low dose steroid therapy for my connective-tissue disorder and the symptoms persist." Ignoring my point about the blurry vision, Dr. Bates counters the steroid argument. "Your current dosage is too low to make a difference," she says with certainty. "But wouldn't I get headaches with migraines?", I ask, my eyes narrowing in undisguised suspicion.

"Not necessarily. It's possible to experience a migraine without the sensation of a headache", she educates me. Though unable to explain the numbness throughout my body, or the sustained blurry vision, she remains adamant in her diagnosis. As much as I want Dr. Bates to be right, my haunting intuition tells me her theory is premature—and that we're dealing with something far more ominous.

Nevertheless, I'm driven to grasp onto something—anything, that offers even the slightest hope of putting an end to these horrendous symptoms. Agreeing to the steroids, I schedule a follow-up appointment in two weeks and leave praying the prescription I clutch will work.

Driving home in the blur that now constitutes my normal vision, I head straight to the pharmacy, anxious to begin treatment immediately. Handing the moist, crumpled slip to the pharmacist to decipher, as I watch him unravel it, I realize how tightly I must have held onto it, almost as though I subconsciously sensed its invaluable properties, or, more likely, tried to will them into it. Aimlessly browsing through the greeting cards as he fills it, my mind is pre-occupied, desperate for this latest treatment to work.

Optimistically, I ingest the first pill. Though I continue to take subsequent ones on schedule, my symptoms remain unchanged. Rationalizing that I haven't given the treatment enough time, I try to suppress my growing discouragement. However, it's impossible to deny the ineffectivity when, by the completion of the regiment, I notice no improvement. Clearly, what's occurring is far more serious than migraines.

And just in case I'm not convinced, my body insidiously drives the point home further, with worsening symptoms over the next few days. I'm overcome with alarm even before opening my eyes Saturday morning, at the realization that the numbness in my left foot has traveled up my entire leg. Nauseated, I again fight the urge to vomit. In an attempt to distract myself, I rub the dry, crusty sleepers out of the corners of my eyes and struggle to decipher the blurry numbered clues of the crossword I started yesterday. But by 10:00 a.m., the symptoms are all-consuming.

Too scared to wait until Monday morning office hours, I sort through my ever-growing stack of doctors' appointment cards, locate the neurologist's, and dial her number. Her partner, Dr. Brown, is on call this weekend and responds immediately. Based on the symptoms I describe, she instructs me to go directly to her office.

Repeating the same exam, the findings remain normal. This just isn't adding up—something is drastically wrong! "Could this be Multiple Sclerosis or a stroke?", I worry out loud. Her intense, thoughtful expression, followed by several moments of silence, tells me she is considering the question I hadn't intentionally asked, but just sort of blurted out. After careful contemplation, she concludes, "Although M.S. can cause visual disturbance and weakness, you definitely didn't have a stroke."

More animated and personable than her partner, I find her far easier to relate to. She tells me about her children, where she lives, and why she moved to her new office. She shares a refreshing, human side of doctors that patients seldom see, but need to know exists. Amid the aura of her down-to-earth attitude, I'm immediately at ease, sharing reciprocal openness and honesty crucial to effective doctor/patient relationships.

Though unable to diagnose based on today's unrevealing exam, my symptoms concern her enough to order a stat EVOKED POTENTIAL TEST, which measures a patient's response time to rapid-succession, visual stimuli. "This is one of the most effective techniques used to rule out M.S.", she anticipates and responds to the obvious question before I verbalize it.

I hate this test! It hurts my eyes to stare incessantly at the black and white checkered screen as flashing impulses are rapidly introduced. The wider I'm asked to open them, the more they ache. I can't wait until it's over. And it doesn't help that the technician, though cordial, remains stoically non-committal. Intellectually, I realize it's her job not to reveal any results—but it's my body. The irony of such discretion is that complete strangers know the direction of my fate before I do. Just as I begin to wonder if it ever will, the test ends and the electrodes are removed from the surface of my head. Looking imploringly into her eyes, I'm frustrated by their blank expression which tells me nothing.

My body desperately aches for sleep. Unfortunately, it aches in other ways as well. Tonight is just awful. Sharp, stabbing, pins-and-needles viciously penetrate deep into my muscles, while intermittent waves of chills cycle through me. Sporadically, various appendages go numb. My right leg is continually weak. I'm afraid to stand up without leaning most of my weight against something, for fear I'll collapse. Unnerved by these symptoms, the potential for devastating results from the M.S. test is undeniable.

I promised my family I would fight whatever this is, and I will. Just looking into their three concerned faces, whose eyes reflect the private, unspoken needs each of them depend on me for, is my incentive. But realistically, is even the most extreme determination, by itself, enough?

Every time the phone rings, I anxiously pick up on the first ring, hoping it's the neurologist with my test results, while at the same time, afraid to hear what she has to say. There is an unmistakable immediacy in my hellos. They are a little too quick, a little too short, to sound natural. I detect disappointment in my own voice after answering expectantly, only to learn it's an unrelated, superfluous call. The "Oh it's you", spoken in an unintentionally lowered, flat tone, leaves my lack of enthusiasm transparent. But the three o'clock phone call is different. This time, it's the doctor with my test results, which registered within normal limits.

Regardless of the unrevealing results, I'm desperately ill. And I don't need a test to convince me of that! My body no longer responds like the one I've known intimately for the last forty-five years. As though I've been transplanted into someone else's, everything about me is different: my inner temperature control mechanism is virtually non-existent, my circulatory, digestive and nervous systems are adversely affected, and, my memory unreliable. My speech is no longer spontaneous, but calculated—and even at that, I never know what I'll unintentionally blurt out next. Whatever happened to that outgoing author, who confidently addressed large audiences, when my first book, "Lupus: My Search for a Diagnosis", was released? Where did this insecure, introverted person—a virtual stranger to me—come from? And what inexplicable phenomenon could cause such a drastic, overnight transformation?

Even the way I interact with my closest friends reflects a difference so extreme—so sudden—it scares me. As I sit with some of them in our local, small town coffee shop, the kind that intoxicates you with the aroma of fresh-perked coffee and artery-clogging bacon sizzling the moment you pull into a parking spot, something feels wrong. With a warm familiarity big cities lack, the waitress pours a cup of decaffeinated coffee for one of the regulars, whose car just pulled up, trusting to memory that this is what he'll want. The hurried attempt to be efficient causes the hot liquid to backsplash against her hand, eliciting a half-whispered expletive. Watching the gentleman appreciatively accept the coffee as he walks into the restaurant, from the outstretched hand of the waitress who has long since regained her composure, I absentmindedly shift my gaze to the white laminated daily specials board. The shiny surface intensifies my blurry vision, rendering the menu impossible to read.

Meanwhile, whiffs of previously enticing diner smells invade my nasal passages without temptation. I don't understand it. Food, up until now, one of my best friends in life—at times too good a friend—no longer has any appeal. What's happening to me that could cause such a basic instinct to be affected so dramatically? As I look around, I realize my appetite isn't the only thing that's different. My personality's changed. Suddenly I'm inexplicably distant from the close friends that surround me, too animated in their own conversations to notice.

Ironically, I first sensed this out-of-character, removed state immediately following the lights' incident, dismissing it as preoccupation. In retrospect, my lack of concern was premature. If anything, the eerie sensation is more pronounced by the day. I no longer feel like one of the regulars. Instead, I'm a stranger enclosed in an invisible bubble, unnervingly distant, both physically and emotionally. I hear bits and pieces of what is being said, I'm vaguely aware of what I'm saying in response, but I feel so faraway. More an observer than a participant, not only am I emotionally distanced from them, physically I perceive myself as further away from the table than anyone else. This is really starting to freak me out!

My friends' images are a blur through my eyes. The more I try to focus on them, the more nauseous I become. Just looking at them across the table makes my stomach queasy. Unlike moments ago, the physical sensation of being too faraway reverses itself. Now I feel like we're touching noses. It produces the same uncomfortable distortion one gets when someone sticks something in front of your face, so near your eyes that you have to move it away before you can focus on it. Complicating breakfast table conversation further is my inability to turn from side to side in an effort to face people speaking to me, without triggering the urge to vomit. Out of necessity, I stare straight ahead.

Though I sit in uncharacteristic silence, I'm a captive prisoner in the confusion of my own mind. An unconvincing replica of my former self, my friends continually try to engage me into the meaningful conversations we once had. But I resist. My mind is far more occupied than they could ever know, but on a plane all its own. The conversation they don't hear is the one I have with myself, as I desperately try to understand what has happened to the me I no longer know.

My friends are becoming suspicious. The frequency and content of their questions demonstrate undisguised alarm over my dramatic and unexplained overnight transformation. "Eileen, are you okay?', they repeatedly ask in voices laced with concern. "Did something happen?" "Is there anything we can do to help?", they offer compassionately. Still unable to come to terms with symptoms and fears my own mind cannot yet comprehend, I tell them I'm fine, unsuccessfully trying to convince myself as much as anyone, as the seeds of denial are planted.

Yet, with each passing day, I'm further and further removed, involuntarily swallowed into my own little world. My lack of appetite is impossible to camouflage, as is the rapid and substantial weight loss that results. I'm unsteady on my feet, have difficulty reading and see the world through dull, blurry eyes, ringed in black. One friend after another observes that I'm just not myself.

As much as they try to understand what happened to me, since the bizarre lights' incident I eventually share, they are as perplexed as I am—except for one friend, who happens to be a psychologist. Throughout the entire breakfast I vaguely sensed her attention to my uncharacteristic demeanor. Even through blurry eyesight, I noticed sincere concern in her eyes. With all the sensitivity a good therapist requires, she gently remarks, "Eileen, your description of a bubble-like, removed sensation is what I frequently hear from my stroke clients. What you're describing is disassociation." The moment the term leaves her lips, my mind transports me back to Psychology 101, where I first heard it. Searching the archives of my memory, I recall enough of the original lecture to realize the validity of her statement. Listening as intently as my la-la land state allows, I'm almost in disbelief over the bombshell-like tidbit discovered in our local coffee shop, where people are on a first name basis and conversation is usually limited to small town gossip. On the other hand, something about the confidence with which she delivers this observation convinces me she really knows her stuff. After gulping down her last swallow of coffee, she offers a final piece of advice on her way out the door. "Try to pay particular attention to your heartbeat. Focusing on its steady rhythm will help you feel more connected."

chapter four

Escalating Fears

Well-intentioned as Eddie's efforts to minimize my fears may be, they backfire as he returns from church with Storey, enthusiastic over our priest's offer to visit. As nonchalantly as possible, no doubt a concerted effort on his part to avoid alarming me, he informs me, "Eileen, I asked Father if he would anoint you and he readily agreed. Just give him a call to let him know when a visit would be convenient." Wait just one minute! Out of the clear blue my husband asks our pastor to make a special trip to our home to bless me and I'm not supposed to worry?

I see right through his matter-of-fact delivery. Eddie's scared, and that scares me. The look in his eyes is incongruous to the casual act he attempts. He sees this move as imperative. It's like he's asking me to receive the sacrament of Last Rites, (generally administered to Roman Catholics on their deathbeds), but that he doesn't want me to know. He realizes the finality of that step would terrify me. On the other hand, to go out of his way to request it, he, too, must suspect I'm dying. No wonder I catch him staring at me with such sad eyes, lately.

My anxiety goes beyond the knot tightening in the pit of my stomach. With one look at my terror-stricken face, which Eddie reads with the accuracy of someone who has had years of practice interpreting its many expressions, he is quick to explain, "Hon, this is NOT the same blessing administered to people who are dying." (Who said he isn't a mind reader?") "Instead", he explains, "you will be receiving the Anointing of the Sick." Listening to him describe it, it sounds precautionary to me—like being blessed in advance, just in case I die. Regardless of his efforts to reassure me by downplaying the purpose of it, I'm not convinced. Undaunted by my skepticism, and driven by the importance he places upon it, he adamantly pursues the subject until I promise to at least consider it.

For reasons I can't comprehend myself yet, within the week my fingers find their way to our priest's phone number. Apprehensively punching in the appropriate digits, before I realize it I'm inviting him to visit our home, the blessing issue still unresolved in my own mind. It it with considerable trepidation that I answer the door to his knock.

Any hesitation I have diminishes in his presence. I welcome the opportunity to voice my deepest fears to this intent listener. When I get to the part of sharing the potential for impending paralysis, I'm speaking from such an inner depth, as I look up into open space, that I almost forget he's here. Lost in the worst case scenario images playing over and over again in my mind, his soft-spoken, almost hypnotic voice gently draws me back to reality.

As his words begin to register, I hear him say, "Eileen, I know you're strong enough to handle whatever comes your way". Asking myself how he could be so sure, I wish I shared his confidence—but I don't. Hopefully, he knows something that I do not. As he anoints me with oil and administers the blessing, I pray he's right.

Even before opening the puffy, large square envelope, I recognize it as a wedding invitation. The feel of the high quality, bonded paper distinguishes it from the other, more mundane mail I receive today. Addressed in fancy, handwritten lettering, as opposed to the computer-generated labels of the rest, the envelope is cushioned, undoubtedly with the white tissue inserts and stamped, smaller response envelope and reply card typically included with wedding invitations.

Though I knew it was coming, receiving it serves as a tangible reminder of a special and exciting time for our family. We have not one, but two, weddings to look forward to within a couple of months of each other. Incredulous as it is to me, my cousin, the one whose Christening I remember to this day—(probably because my aunt was so animated that finally, after three daughters, she had a son)—is getting married next week. His fiance, someone he's dated for years, is a girl the entire family has readily grown to love. That part was easy—she couldn't be nicer or more natural, the kind of person who seems like she was always a part of the family. My cousin deserves someone special. Considerate and soft-spoken, his sensitivity to others reminds me of his dad's, who just happens to be a favorite uncle of mine.

I'm looking forward to their wedding because I believe in them as a couple. For every kind and warm gesture my cousin initiates, his fiance is equally thoughtful. They exude love not only to one another but to those around them, as well. Just the thought of their up-and-coming marriage transforms my face into a broad and genuine smile. Unfortunately, it is short-lived. With comparable spontaneity, my cheeks deflate back to normal, my previously upbeat expression replaced by a grim, tight-lipped response to momentary anxiety as I struggle to read today's mail through blurry vision.

Setting the bills aside, I open the invitation first. As anticipated, it is to my brother's wedding—the brother who, as a young child, cried inconsolably when his only sister got married and left home. Ironically, now it's big sister's turn to cry. Generating my tears will be mixed emotions: disbelief that the child I once took care of is an adult, capable of fathering and caring for a child of his own—and genuine happiness in that he fell in love with such a wonderful person. If ever I could picture him with a soul mate, she's the one. They even resemble one another. More importantly, their love for each other is written all over the special looks they reserve exclusively for one another.

As my mind reflects on their relationship, it resurrects a touching scene from last Christmas Eve which, like every one since Stacey was born, was celebrated at our home. The atmosphere is Christmas-shop festive, with white twinkling lights aglow throughout the downstairs. They, and the crackling fire, are intentionally the only form of illumination, casting a soft, romantic glow throughout. Christmas songs playing in the background add to the mood. By the time one of my favorites comes on, "The Christmas Bell that Couldn't Jingle", it is drowned out by the excited voices of family members opening gifts. Shrills of delight emanate with the discovery of items at the top of their wish lists, (which though they longed for, couldn't count on getting). Then there are a few surprises and the inevitable annual atrocities one learns to tactfully accept with convincing appreciation, only to return, store indefinitely, or give away later to someone who, hopefully, will find it more appealing.

Still carrying my eggnog-spiced Kahlua with whipped cream and chocolate shavings, a December tradition in our household, I enter our bedroom to up the volume of the music, only to unexpectedly come upon my brother and sister-in-law-to-be in a loving embrace. Staring intently into one another's large, dark almond eyes, stunning features of each, they're so engrossed in themselves, and undoubtedly caught up in the festivity of the season—evidenced by the gifts they obviously exchanged privately, judging from the torn wrapping paper still strewn about, they're unaware of my presence. Choosing not to interrupt their special moment, (certainly I can listen to my song later), I concertedly back my way soundlessly out of the room, grateful for the thick carpet which made me successfully oblivious to two people lost in their own private world of love. If I read them right, this is a Christmas they'll remember forever—and the start of many more.

Ironically, it wasn't long ago, less than a few years, when this brother spent almost every Saturday night at our house. He and Eddie would stay awake watching games hours after I'd fallen asleep, only to be startled awake by their loud cheering or, more often than not, spontaneous shouting at individual players or, the team as a whole, exasperated by their impression of a less than optimal performance. It must be a male thing. They seem convinced that if one yells loud enough in the direction of the television screen, the players will hear and respond by improving their play and, ultimately, winning the game. Lest you doubt this theory, I challenge you to walk into any sport's bar and see for yourself.

At any rate, these Saturday night "dates", as we affectionately referred to them, took place for years. When I grocery shopped, I automatically planned on him for dinner. But suddenly, everything changed. His visits became few and far between. His dates were now real. Long before he admitted to it, we realized he'd fallen in love. It was written all over his face and dictated his dramatic change in lifestyle. And it was good. Good for him because he was so happy—and good for me because once I'd met and gotten to know her, I realized how lucky I was to be gaining such a sensitive sister-in-law. Life is good.

Wrapping my cousin's wedding gift evokes feelings of excitement and nostalgia. It also unleashes underlying, but none-the-less unmistakable anxiety. Will I physically be able to handle this very special day they've dreamt of most of their lives? I feel so weak, not to mention exhausted, having been up most of the night due to swallowing difficulty. Yet I'm determined to be there. This is one wedding I don't want to miss!

The church they selected is familiar to us. As a matter-of-fact, it's one of our favorites, traditional and ornate, like the ones we grew up belonging to, in contrast to the more modern and starker designs constructed today. Unfortunately, with its authenticity comes the immense staircase erected during an age when handicapped access wasn't a consideration in building. Precariously, I ascend, leaning most of my weight on Eddie, as we painstakingly and conspicuously approach the entrance. Once inside, I admire the massive and detailed Corinthian columns, delicate-featured, pastel painted statues and beautiful stained glass windows whose intensity peaks with the bright sun's rays shining on them—all of which seem more impressive to me with every successive visit to this breathtakingly memorable place of worship.

Interrupting my visual journey of this true work of art, my attention is diverted to the back of the church as ushers roll the traditional white carpet down the aisle and the music begins. Thoughtfully, the bride, looking not surprisingly stunning on her day, included all three of my cousin's sisters as attendants. It's just further testimony of the considerate person she is.

From the altar, the groom looks expectant and emotional as he focuses on her slow but deliberate approach toward him. As the pleasant aroma of the beautiful flowers invades my nostrils, my thoughts reflect on the observation that they look as sure about the imminent vows they will momentarily make as any couple I've ever seen. I silently pray that they will always share the unmistakable love evident in their eyes and hearts today, while at the same time I thank God that Eddie and I are so in love. As they exchange their vows, Eddie's warm hand reaches over for mine, his gentle squeeze reminding me that he, too, is silently renewing our own.

With the conclusion of their beautiful ceremony, we follow the bride and groom, along with the rest of the congregation, to the receiving line at the entrance of the church. From what seems like a faraway distance, I hear my newest cousin tease, "Eileen, do you mean to tell me we got all dressed up for you and you walked right by us without even noticing?". Incredulously, she's right. In my trance-like state, I walked right by the bride and groom, oblivious to their presence, which, consequently, I failed to acknowledge. Though I laugh on the outside over the embarrassing oversight others interpret as pre-occupation with the rest of the guests, and being caught up in the ambiance of the moment, inside I'm scared. It's like I'm not even here, or that a part of me is separated from the rest of the group, yet, in reality, I'm physically surrounded by them. As I leave the church, I silently implore God to guide my physicians in their search for an explanation to the dramatic and inexplicable change I've undergone—and, more importantly, to help me recover.

Seated at a table with guests of the bride, it doesn't take Eddie and I long to warm up to these people we're meeting for the first time. They're all so friendly. As waitresses in black skirts and white shirts duck out of each other's way as they pour champagne into sparkling glasses to the right of plates whose mirror-like shine reflect our own images back at us, we get to know the other guests. Somewhat surprised, I soon learn that my current medical status is not the secret I thought it was, and that others are aware of it through the grapevine.

One person in particular, an occupational therapist seated to my immediate left, reaches out to me in a way I'll never forget. After tactfully ascertaining I'm comfortable discussing it, she inquires further regarding my current condition. When I allude to swallowing difficulty, which remains a mystery to me, she nods knowingly—as though I'm not the first to complain of this symptom. Apparently many of her stroke patients experience this alarming sensation. I'm appreciative when she demonstrates a chin-to-chest position to assume when it is at its worst, particularly when my momentary experimentation with it results in immediate relief. Though I expected to leave the reception having gained a new cousin, I had no way of predicting the warm acquaintances I made and invaluable medical advice I received.

Without warning, intense, excruciating headaches, deep throughout my entire head, begin to occur. Lasting approximately five to twenty minutes, I have several throughout the day and night, preventing sleep, or even a semblance of everyday functioning. Unnerved by their severity, I'm afraid to drive, and do so infrequently.

Beginning with a prickly sensation, within minutes it escalates to unmistakable pain. It hurts to lie on the affected spot and, at times, there is a trickling sensation around the site. Associated with pins-and-needles, or novocaine-like numbness on the unrelated side of my face, it seems that the side opposite the headache location is where most symptoms occur. Periodically, one eye tears uncontrollably. Occasionally, a pulling sensation forces one open wider than the other. Sometimes I drool from the corner of my mouth. At other times, my lips are unnaturally askew.

Terrified by the new and more frightening symptoms which develop by the day, I covertly begin a journal to my family, though I have no intention of them reading it—at least not yet.

Dear Family:

It's so hard for me to write this letter to you. I can barely see the print through the warm, salty tears which bathe my cheeks, cooling as they journey down my face, leaving their streaky, tell-tale trails behind. But there are things that must be said.

It is 2:30 a.m. and, once again, sleep is out of the question. Preventing it are the physical and, to-date, inexplicable symptoms I've experienced since the two multi-faceted lights' episodes ten weeks ago. Those cascading, seemingly-harmless clear bubbles have created untold havoc in my body. I don't feel like the same person—I'm clearly NOT the same person. Something changed, dramatically, in me that day. I hardly know myself anymore. I feel as though the mind and personality of someone foreign to me has taken up residency in the familiar shell of my old body. And even that shell changes daily, before my disbelieving eyes.

For starters, I can't explain the out-of-character, non-existent appetite trigger responsible for my alarmingly rapid weight loss. The bony configuration of ribs, prominent enough to easily count even through blurry vision, ominously reflects back at me as I get out of the bathtub. Scared into denial, I spontaneously avert my eyes from the mirror, but not soon enough to miss my significantly reduced waistline, leaving me unable to escape more frightening by the day reality.

And who is this person who dissolves into tears, repeatedly, for no apparent reason? Certainly not the wife and mother you've known in the past. I'm so scared over what's insidiously tormenting my health that I can barely face you, the people I love most, without undisguised terror written all over me. This nightmare, from which fate refuses to allow me to awaken, can only be fully understood by the person living it.

My eyes ache relentlessly, too painful to touch and too blurry to make sustained reading possible. Dull and dark-circled, I barely recognize them. Frighteningly, the numbness in my lips, tongue, face, feet, legs and hands continues, awakening me to the unnerving sensation of at least one novocaine-numb appendage. The episodic pain in my head is far more severe than the worst headache I've ever had in my life, re-defining my definition of the word terror.

Though I've been trying to get medical help since the onset, I'm spinning my wheels, continually imploring reluctant physicians to initiate further investigation.

I'm scheduled to see Dr. Bates tomorrow. I intend to tell her that based on the ineffectivity of the migraine treatment she recommended, she grossly underestimated the gravity of my condition. My fear is that without more immediate aggressive medical intervention, including repeated brain scans and round-the-clock observation, irreparable neurological damage can occur. My desperation to avoid that is all-consuming.

Yet, at a time when I've never felt so sick in my life—far more ill than when hospitalized in the past—my physicians don't see admission as warranted. But doctors can be wrong. I just pray Dr. Bates isn't.

I love you all.

Mom

"Dr. Bates, the trial with high dose steroids proved futile. My symptoms continue more aggressively than ever. I now get severe headaches, not to mention muscles that involuntarily jerk and twitch", I report assertively. Sitting on the exam table as she observes my muscles to the background noise of the disposable, white paper sheet crinkling, she remarks, "I see absolutely no evidence of inappropriate muscle activity".

Visualizing the needle on an imaginary blood pressure meter soaring in my mind, I hear myself think that that's not surprising, since these symptoms occur transiently. Is it any wonder why they're so hard to diagnose?

Feeling somewhat like a person whose car repeatedly won't start, only to have it rev up immediately for the mechanic when he arrives with his tow truck, I listen anxiously as Dr. Bates thinks aloud. Smugly commenting, "Once again your neurological findings are normal—As expected, I see no evidence of anything physically wrong". Familiar anger pulsates through my veins, igniting me from head-to-toe, when she questions "How is your personal life? Have you been depressed lately?". In my mind, I'm thinking: "How can you be so obtuse? At the moment my emotional state is normal, but it won't be for long if physicians such as yourself continue to refuse to recognize the validity of this illness and institute appropriate treatment—immediately!"

Frustrating as it is, her question comes as no surprise. I've come across this attitude before, where the inflated egos of a segment of physicians interfered with their ability to consider the potential for serious illness unless they were able to diagnose it themselves. It scares me to think how many trusting, unsuspecting patients have lost their lives to such medical overconfidence. Unwilling to once again subject myself as a victim of any doctor's out-of-control self-esteem, by allowing what I'm convinced is a serious neurological condition to remain undetected, I intend to fight back as diligently as if my life depends on it—for all I know, it may.

"I don't know what other words to use to convey to you that something physical, not emotional, occurred the day I saw those lights.

Whatever it was, it has dramatically impacted my entire nervous system." As a result of my persistence, and out of exasperation that she makes no meaningful connections, she reluctantly agrees to refer me to a neurologist at a large teaching hospital.

In a follow-up letter to my primary care physician, she describes me as demonstrating "normal, intact speech, language and cognition", but comments that I appear "anxious". I can almost feel my blood pressure rise as I read her poor attempt at psychological analysis, something she isn't trained to do—and it shows. How unfortunate she's unable to recognize my reaction as normal and empathize with how it must feel, overnight, to develop such alarming symptoms, instead of impulsively jumping to inaccurate conclusions. In contrast, Dr. Michaels is extremely sensitive to the frightening ramifications associated with this inexplicable condition. Why is it so difficult for other physicians to put themselves in their patients' shoes?

As Dr. Bates's letter continues, she states, "Eileen denies any significant stress except for concern over her current symptoms". She, however, adamantly adheres to her theory that the condition is probably due to stress or depression, in the absence of anything physical. Notating that I was "vehemently unreceptive" to this inference, the letter ends informing him of the teaching hospital referral.

Journal Entry #2

Dear Eddie:

When the going gets rough, it's comforting to know I can always reach out to my best friend, and that you'll be there. Regretfully, this is one of those times there is nothing you can do other than listen. Somehow, just the thought that you're there for that, at such an uncertain time, is reassuring. I can't find the words to do justice to a kind of sick I never knew existed until now, yet insidiously defies diagnosis. The inexplicable and grossly abnormal sensations throughout my body, most particularly the pins-and-needles and numbness, send fears of impending paralysis up and down my spine. The terror elicited by this thought, alone, leaves me frantically trying to communicate with you and the girls while I can.

I feel scared and cheated. I've never in my life felt as tormented as in the last three and a half months. I can barely look at you, Stacey and Storey without bursting into tears. I'm so angry over this undesirable situation over which I have no control.

And the medical profession's lack of compassion doesn't make it any easier. Since the onset of this sudden, life-altering nightmare, too many physicians have grossly underestimated the severity of what has occurred. From being brushed off until doctors return from vacation, to hearing it isn't anything serious, to being told I'm experiencing migraines, I'm getting nowhere fast. My pleas for hospitalization for the purpose of observation are dismissed with the rationale that insurance would never approve the cost. Given advice to do something "fun" for the weekend, I'm told to just relax, meaningless words uttered by doctors who don't have a clue as to what they're asking.

Angrily, I'm informed that I've had $9,000.00 worth of unnecessary testing just to learn that I'm fine. Well, I'm telling you I'm not fine! I don't care if I've had nine million dollars worth of testing, something devastating has happened within my body—and I'm terrified!

Love,
Eileen

chapter five
University Expertise?

Parents' Weekend couldn't have coincided with more spectacular weather—sunny and crisp days, with cool, sleep-inducing nighttime temperatures. High on a hill, overlooking breathtaking Lake Cayuga, surrounded by Fall foliage at its peak, the view from Stacey's dorm room is breathtakingly indescribable. Getting there is another story. Steep flights of stairs, the only access to the majority of her beautiful but cliff-like campus, are situated, out of necessity, throughout.

Observing other baby boomer parents huff and puff, I feel less self-conscious of my own struggle to get from one event to the next, none of which are in close proximity of each other. But I'm determined to take an active role in this weekend. From the homemade cookies I bake, to attending the President's welcome dinner, to seeing a play, meeting other parents, viewing sporting events, admiring the beautiful colored-light lit fountains each night and attending the movie of the week, we do it all. But more importantly, we share quality time with our daughter, whom we've both missed tremendously.

Fun as it is, I find myself feeling insecure, subtly evidenced only by Eddie and me as I cling tighter to banisters, stay closer to him at all times, and count the hours until I'm able to lie down. By the end of the weekend, we leave fulfilled having seen how effectively Stacey has adjusted to college life, yet sharing health concerns that Eddie and I intentionally managed to camouflage from her. The busy schedule and countless distractions were conducive to our goal. We want her to concentrate on her studies—not worry about her mom's health.

The remaining two week wait for the much-anticipated university appointment drags out agonizingly. An undeniable increase in the frequency and severity of the now-daily headaches makes me more conscious of every minute. Previous forms of distraction have become ineffective in coping with the intense pain. While blurry vision prevents sustained reading, making it impossible to lose myself in a good book, even crossword puzzles, my only escape during the isolated and involuntarily wide awake midnight-to-dawn hours, are no longer realistic. Half the time the blanks I attempt to fill in don't correspond to the numbered clues I try to solve for. Sevens look like ones, and sixes like eights, through my visual distortion.

Pins-and-needles mercilessly ignore no part of my body, with their injection-like stabbing deeper and more forceful than ever. Per usual, my lips are excessively dry and colorless and, at times, numb. The numbness often spreads to the inside of my mouth. My tongue feels uncharacteristically thick and I have swallowing difficulty so pronounced I'm fearful of choking. Nauseated twenty-four hours a day, large stores are a problem to negotiate, with depth perception irregularity intensified by the high ceilings.

Recently, while experiencing a tipping sensation, I toppled into the shelves of a grocery aisle, noisily knocking canned goods to the floor. (Embarrassed by the attention it attracted, judging from the number of people gawking as I self-consciously attempted to right myself, I experienced, firsthand, how uninvolved members of our society can be. No one asked if I was okay or needed assistance.)

The incident played on my own guilt as I asked myself if I, too, out of convenience and/or lack of assertiveness ever looked the other way rather than helping someone in need—and I didn't like my answer. But I learned a valuable lesson that day.

Further reflection is interrupted by excruciating muscle pain nothing alleviates. I feel like I have constant charley horses in my legs. The last time I drove, my hands were so tingly grasping the steering wheel, I worried I could lose all feeling. Frightened for my own safety, and that of my passengers, (especially the student carpool I transport), I make the necessary but regrettable decision to cease driving. The risks far outweigh any reluctance to relinquish my independence. Hopefully I'll be able to reverse this decision once we get whatever is occurring under control.

With my appendages jerking involuntarily, buzzing sounds in my ears, and a periodic metallic taste in my mouth, (reminiscent of a flavor of childhood, when I remember sucking on my brother's toy silver guns, from his little black holster with shiny studs), I cannot dismiss the probability of a neurological problem. Nor do I see how any physician could.

With the orange floss, clothespin worry doll Storey made me tucked in my pocket, I say good-bye to my family as they leave for work and school. The hug Eddie and I share is a little closer—a little more intense, than usual, reflecting our unspoken hope for today's visit.

Shortly, my mother and aunt arrive to drive me to my appointment. The intense discomfort in my head, coupled with the unrelenting nausea and dizziness which plagues me throughout the ride, only serves to further confirm the necessity of this visit—as if I needed confirmation!

Armed with the requested x-rays, scans and medical records accumulated since being diagnosed with connective-tissue disease twelve years ago, I enter the neurologist's office. As I sit facing him, he meticulously reads through my records, periodically questioning things requiring clarification. But, for the most part, there is awkward silence as he scans. At one point, I volunteer information regarding recent symptoms. His halfhearted response, barely audible and uttered with his eyes never leaving my chart, conveys to me that he prefers to give the notes his undivided attention. Acting on his cue, I sit quietly, visually taking in everything in the sparse, walk-in-closet sized exam room, within seconds: the blood pressure cuff hanging sloppily from the wall, the paper covered examining table, a small sink, a table which doubles as his desk, two chairs, florescent lights, a four drawer file cabinet and a Norman Rockwell print on the wall across from me. The longer I stare at these same objects, the more boring they become. By the time my eyes dance from one to the other for what seems like the hundredth time, I'm seriously regretting that I didn't think to bring an activity. As though reading my mind, his forty-five minute review of my records concludes.

Sitting back in his chair, stretching out his short legs to their maximum, he peaks his hands together, tepee-style, against his pursed lips and scrutinizes me. After an awkward and prolonged silence, a barrage of questions ensues, including whether I cry often, sleep well, have a good appetite, demonstrate normal energy and have friends.

I answer his questions honestly, "I don't cry often, I have trouble sleeping since the onset of symptoms associated with the lights' incident and, of late, my appetite is uncharacteristically non-existent". Acknowledging a slight decrease in energy, I attribute it to my recent lack of sleep. "And yes, I have lots of friends".

His neurological exam blatantly contrasts the others. To begin with, I remain fully dressed. Secondly, it is conducted in a hurried manner. For example, he passes a scent so abruptly under my nostrils, my brain doesn't have time to register and identify it. However, when he repeats the test more slowly, at my request, I easily detect the pleasant aroma of peppermint.

Surprisingly, his exam is the least comprehensive I've had. I would expect just the opposite from a university hospital. I'm given no long and short term memory tests and the entire exam is over within three minutes.

At the conclusion, he smugly informs me, "There's nothing neurologically wrong with you. I suggest you find a good psychiatrist and get on a strong anti-depressant—immediately. And don't bother coming back to see me unless you develop a neurological problem in the future, because you certainly don't have one now!".

If this were a few years ago, my cheeks would still be stinging from his unexpected emotional slap in the face. Once recovered, as much as I might have disagreed with what he was saying, I probably would've played the passive patient role, looked unquestioningly into this doctor-god's eyes and responded, "Yes, doctor". But no more. I've experienced far too much ineptitude on the part of the medical profession, between errors mis-diagnosing my case and that of others, to trust their opinions indisputably. Like them, I'm educated and equipped with my own powers of observation—and I intend to use them. Inarguably convinced neurological involvement resulted from those lights, I intend to pursue the treatment I need.

Unlike my doctors, this is happening to me, personally. Only I know how it feels to live this insidious war raging inside me. And who else stands to suffer irreparable consequences if the physicians I consult guess wrong? I owe it to myself to challenge the medical profession to respect my observations. I can't afford to waste time with doctors who refuse to acknowledge the gravity of my symptoms.

As I get up to leave, I emphatically state disagreement with his assessment of my case. "You're wrong! Something neurological IS going on." Walking out the door, I'm suddenly struck by the realization that his mind was made up before he touched me—consequently, the reason for the rushed, superficial exam. While I'm proud of myself for standing my ground in the face of what, in the past, would've been intimidating opposition, this visit was clearly a waste of time. With self esteem intact, but troubled by my lack of answers, I walk out to the waiting room—to the expectant and hopeful eyes of my mother and aunt.

Initially stunned as I regurgitate his analysis, once it registers, I have to all but physically restrain them from telling him off. And I can't blame them. For too long, they've helplessly witnessed someone they love change, in an inexplicable and negative way, right before their disbelieving eyes. Not only do I look different, I act different. I'm inarguably not the same person they've known for forty-four years, and, like me, they're scared. The car takes on an eerie silence on the way home, with each of us absorbed in the privacy of our own unspoken thoughts. From my perspective, I'm desperate—and a major avenue just fell through. I have no idea where to turn next.

Lying down after my grueling morning excursion, the symptoms are intolerable. My head hurts so badly, I know of no adjective to do justice to the pain. Deep muscle aches in my legs make them almost impossible to move. My mouth, lips and cheeks are novocaine-numb. I feel sick to my stomach, but nowhere near as sick as when momentarily stunned by the warm, wet feeling signifying the involuntary and sustained leakage of urine. My God, I can't go on like this! I need help.

Out of desperation, I call a well-known hospital in a neighboring state where, coincidentally, my mother has an appointment scheduled for the end of the week. Upon hearing my symptoms, a nurse in the Neurology Department recommends that I see their top neurologist. Unfortunately, his first available appointment is two and a half weeks away, which, at the moment, seems like an eternity.

Hearing the concern and urgency in my trembling voice, the nurse suggests an alternative. She advises scheduling the available appointment but, in the interim, showing up at their walk-in day clinic. By going to the clinic, she assures me, "You'll still have the benefit of our state-of-the-art neurological department. The neurologist on call that day will automatically be paged for you". Though she concedes that it isn't as good as having an actual appointment, she points out that "It's a foot in the door". Desperate, and with no other plan at the moment, I decide to follow her suggestion, and go to the day clinic on Friday, while my mom is at her own appointment.

It's a blurry 11:34 p.m. on the digital clock. I can't sleep because of the unnerving sensations throughout my body. The stabbing pins-and-needles are predominantly on my left side tonight. The soles of my feet tingle so much they feel like they're crawling. My head hurts and I'm nauseated. Severe abdominal cramping defies me to even try to rest the weight of my arm against my mid-section. With each cramp, waves of body-wrenching chills are dispersed throughout me.

Tonight's symptoms frighten me more than usual. They last longer and seem more intense. Motivated by fear, and reluctant to be alone, I seek the proximity of Eddie and Storey, whose voices I follow to the family room. To the sounds of their animated discussion over the television show they're watching, I feel more secure just being around them, and elect not to mention my current physical state.

Impatiently, I count the days until our out-of-state medical excursion. In the interim, I manage to get my hands on a letter of paramount interest to me: the latest neurologist's written assessment to Dr. Bates. Beyond disbelief, my anger rises like mercury in a flu patient's thermometer, intensifying by the line, as I read the physical check points he claims to have addressed in his exam. In truth, I spend more time reading his deceptively impressive, lengthy dissertation, than I did on the examining table. With each line, I'm more sickened by the reality of how much power his position wields. His letter inaccurately portrays an exam that was far less comprehensive than he describes, taking credit for procedures he never did. But it's my word against his. As the patient, I'm clearly at the disadvantage.

Even before plowing through the wordy documentation, I detected a hint of bias when he addressed Dr. Bates by his first name. This familiarity implies some degree of friendship between the two physicians, in my mind jeopardizing the chances of an objective opinion. When he goes on to thank the doctor for his referral to evaluate my migraine "hallucinations", I feel my eyes roll from exasperation. This statement speaks volumes. For one, the new doctor is automatically pre-dispositioned to associate my problem with migraines. Secondly, according to my Selectronic's WordFinder, synonyms for hallucination include: delusion, insanity, derangement, aberration and craziness. Is there any doubt where this is going?

Further along, he comments that I "deny crying on a continual basis", nor do I feel an overwhelming urge to cry. He describes me as a "rigid, intelligent person who has picked up a lot of "medicalese" over the years". I can understand how I impressed him as rigid, as I mentally replay the assertive way in which I informed him that my problem is physical, not emotional. Regarding my medical vocabulary, there is no doubt that being a long-term patient provides an education in itself. Contrary to the neurologist, I see this as positive, if not life-saving.

What I've learned goes far beyond medical terminology. I no longer ingest medication on command, like some patient-robot. Instead, I ask what it is, why it is being given, what it can do to improve my condition and, whether it has any deleterious side effects. On more than one occasion, I've refused unfamiliar-looking medication presented to me in a hospital setting, only to find out it was, in fact, the wrong pill and intended for someone else. Patients owe it to themselves to be informed consumers!

With anger that continues to build as I read further, my disbelieving eyes focus on words that never should've been printed. I'm speechless when I get to the part where he suggests my low dose steroids may be "affecting my psyche". Considering I've been on them for ten years without negative psychological side affects, his explanation strikes me as a pathetic rationalization for his lack of competence in establishing an accurate medical diagnosis. He recommends decreasing the already insignificant, 15mg. every-other-day dosage I currently take.

Giving even more credibility to the psychosomatic explanation, he justifies the numbness in my mouth and tongue, as well as the tingling limbs, as symptoms generating from anxiety over my medical condition. Granted, hyperventilation can produce symptoms such as these. Unfortunately, so can far more serious conditions. As a former Lamaze childbirth instructor, I'm very familiar with detecting the signs of hyperventilation and I'm definitely not hyperventilating. Nor does this neurologist, with his neatly laid out psychological scenario that transcends the limits of his medical training, mention ever having observed me hyperventilate.

The conclusion of his letter documents what he conveyed to me in the office, that there is no neurological involvement and I should see a psychiatrist, immediately, for a strong antidepressant. How can anyone, even a doctor with a specialty in neurology, be that sure of himself? I'm reporting serious symptoms—and he's telling me they don't exist! What if he's wrong? Or is his ego too inflated to even entertain that possibility? And more importantly, can he afford not to, when dealing with someone's life?

In a condescending final statement, he acknowledges that I didn't agree with his diagnosis, but that I'm "an intelligent woman he suspects will come around after giving it more thought". When Hell freezes over! What a pompous attitude. And to think, he had the stupidity to put it in writing. It is physicians such as this that destroy credibility toward the medical profession, in general.

Ironically, just when I'm convinced I can barely get through another day of these horrendous symptoms, they insidiously intensify. Beyond a doubt, the sole reason I have any sanity left, as a result of this living nightmare, is due to the ongoing support of family and friends. Their determination, alone, refuses to let me stop fighting what, to date, appears to be a losing battle.

To compensate for my reluctant but necessary decision to temporarily stop driving, while at the same time sensitive to the fact that the cozy, but dimly-lit coffee shop is difficult on my eyes, my friends now "take-out" breakfast to my home. Only instead of meeting once a week, as in the past, they are here daily. That change, in itself, considering their hectic work and family schedules, leaves their own grave fears concerning my health as transparent as if they verbalized the words they intentionally bite their tongues to hold back—as fear they can't possibly hide registers in their faces. The truth is, their ineffectively concealed reactions tell me nothing I don't already know.

As the recipient of their unwavering dedication, I don't know where they find the strength to persevere under such adverse conditions. Yet, like clockwork, the sizzling, flattened hard roll, (which most resembles the kind my friend Debbie and I loved in college and have been unable to duplicate since), is delivered piping hot to this vaguely suggestive representation of the friend they once knew. With the rapid and substantial weight loss, pasty skin, and black-circled, sparkless eyes, I'm hardly recognizable as the person they've shared so many milestones with over the years.

Appearance aside, I don't act like that same friend, as I sit across from them shivering under an afghan, barely able to get down a bite, lost in a distant, removed stare, adding little-to-nothing to their conversation. Not to be discouraged, at least on the surface, they talk to me about anything and everything in a futile effort to re-ignite my former spark. As much as they encourage me to share my feelings, I can't find words dynamic enough to begin to describe what it feels like to become a stranger to yourself—overnight.

With concerted efforts to demonstrate tact, my friends elude to the fact that I don't look like myself. Well-intentioned as their protective use of discretion may be, the inescapable truth is far less considerate, hiding nothing, whenever I look into a mirror. Taken aback by my own reflection, denial convinces me that this can't be me. Instead, some pathetic person stares back through dull, blurry, sparkless eyes. Dressed in clothes that hang off of her like oversized hand-me-downs, her face rarely smiles, but frequently registers pain, evidenced by its contorted winces.

A few friends who are strong enough to level with me, admit I look so bad it scares them. The unspoken thought, that they have legitimate reason to be scared, and that I certainly am, reflects a deep, private fear I'm not able to verbalize to them—yet. For the first time in my life, I'm convinced I'm dying. I can't think of any other explanation for how desperately ill I feel. Unfortunately, my doctors don't yet realize the gravity of my situation. Somehow, I've got to get through to them—my life depends on it.

Waking to the sound of birds chirping excitedly, I lie in bed listening to nature speak. As the balmy Fall breeze blows its unseasonably warm breath in my direction, I consider the analogy of this form of communication to eavesdropping on a conversation spoken in a foreign language I never studied. Though I know meaningful messages surround me, I haven't a clue as to what they're saying. Envying the carefree, primitive existence of my feathered friends, non-intrusively aware of it from the comfort of my bed, I reflect on the contrast between their lives and mine. A fiercely developing headache snaps me back to my inescapable reality.

As my friend's youngest child answers the phone, proudly demonstrating her recently-acquired skill, I can hear the excitement in her voice. The unmistakable sound of a dropped receiver, as its reverberating bounces echo in my ear, is followed by her loudly informing family members that she "got it". When she returns, she recognizes my voice and begins to converse excitedly. Though my response lacks its usual enthusiasm when talking to this little girl I've grown to love, she seems oblivious. Fortunately, Sara's excitement is typical of that of a young child, revolving around her own little world, undaunted by my inability to share her exuberance.

Clearly, I didn't call to talk to Sara today. I'm desperate to speak to her mom, who happens to be one of my closest friends. Since she works full-time, I rely on phone conversations to keep her informed. My out-of-character inattentiveness to her child is due to pre-occupation, as I mentally search for the right words to ask my friend, Sue, for the biggest favor I've ever requested. By the time Sara relinquishes the phone to her, I still haven't found them.

The sound of her voice makes further rehearsal unnecessary. With the spontaneity characteristic of communication between close friends, I drop the tough front reserved for others and disclose my fears, uncensored, to someone I know will understand. "Sue, with the sharp, stabbing pins-and-needles throughout my body, there's obviously nerve involvement. I'm scared that I may end up paralyzed!" At the mere mention of the word, I burst into tears. Between sobs, I continue, "My arms, legs, mouth and tongue go numb everyday. I'm terrified that this means I could lose all sensation, including the ability to communicate. You've got to listen carefully to what I have to say before it's too late", I implore.

This conversation can't be easy for her. I interrupt her efforts to comfort me, telling her "I have to get this out". With tears streaming down my face, the product of love only a mother knows, I express fears of not being here for my daughters, at least not in the capacity they're accustomed to. "You've got to promise if anything happens to me, you will be. I'd do it for you if, God forbid, the tables were turned."

By this time fighting her own emotions, due to the sensitivity of our conversation, her barely audible response, "I know you would", is spoken with sincerity. As uncomfortable as this is for both of us, I can't drop it yet, not until I'm sure she understands the entire picture of what I'm asking. Continuing, I request that she "Be there for the important times in their lives". Squeezing my eyes shut tightly, I fight tears so profuse, I can barely get out, "For the mom things". She promises me, as I dissolve into tears the moment I verbalize the heart-wrenching request, that "I know exactly what you mean and you can count on me—but, hopefully, that will never be necessary". With that assurance, our sad, but necessary conversation, which reached a depth of our friendship never before explored, concluded.

Throughout this entire nightmare, my friends continue the early morning, weekday breakfasts, delivered steaming hot and cooked to order. More importantly, they provide an opportunity for intense conversations, in which I share my deepest fears—that I'm dying. The tears misting in their eyes confirm that they, too, suspect this grim probability. I look sicker by the day, a fact they're upfront about. The lack of pretense in our relationship is what makes me respect it most. As I sit and talk to them, I layer myself with afghans to help counteract the waves of chills surging through my body. While I cover up goosebumps, with enough clothing to survive in Siberia, there are aspects of this illness that I can't possibly hide.

My friends tell me my eyes have lost their spark and look duller by the day, as the raccoon-like rings circling them grow darker. And their observations don't end there. They can't help but notice my non-existent appetite, I barely touch my breakfasts. At times, I start to fall asleep while talking to them, only to awaken abruptly with the onset of my next headache. To help compensate for swallowing difficulty, I suck lemon drops incessantly. Always, I look at these friends I love through blurry vision. At times, I feel so removed and detached from their conversations. My once similar lifestyle now contrasts theirs', dramatically. Previously as happy and cheerful as they, since that inexplicable light show I'm sick and terrified—and nothing they do or say takes that unsettling feeling away.

For as concerned as my friends are, Eddie is understandably more devastated by the dramatic and overnight changes he witnesses in disbelief. Fear engulfs him, unmistakably registered in his intense, out-of-character sad eyes as he helplessly observes my color turn pasty white at the onset of each excruciating headache, while blood-shot eyes connect with his concerned ones—the transparency of my own bewilderment and terror reflected back at him. I'm weak to the point that, at times, he has to support me. When I do manage to get some well-overdue sleep, it is only by sitting up uncomfortably straight, in an effort to counteract the ever-constant swallowing difficulty which, when lying down, creates an unnerving choking sensation.

My muscles jerk involuntarily, startling Eddie out of a sound sleep from the impact of the affected limb's vibration against our mattress. In addition to the fear associated with this abnormal occurrence, I regret his sleep disruption. As the sole breadwinner, he works extra long days to help compensate for my loss of salary. Uncomplainingly, he reaches the point of exhaustion, day after day, and though he deserves an uninterrupted night's sleep, he seldom gets it. Yet, every morning he manages to repeat the same process, and cheerfully, at that. Hopefully, this book will amount to a respectable effort on my part, as I take advantage of turning a negative experience positive, (while at the same time affording myself a healthy distraction), to thank him in a small way for all that he does for me and our girls.

My reflection on Eddie's industrious qualities is unexpectedly interrupted when walking barefoot into the bathroom I realize the ceramic tile floor isn't cold, as it customarily is, twelve months a year. Once again, my faulty temperature control mechanism is blatantly resurrected to my awareness, just when I'd succeeded in putting it out of my mind for a few hours. At the same time, my right arm begins to go numb. As the words on the glossy surface of the prescription insert I attempt to read run together in one big, continuous blur, impossible to decipher, I lose my balance, catching myself on the sink.

Too scared by these increasingly serious symptoms to remain emotionally supportive but medically helpless a moment longer, two weeks prior to my appointment Eddie calls the neurologist I'm scheduled to see. I can hear nervousness in a stoic voice he seldom exhibits as he methodically details my symptoms to Dr. Johnson. The purpose of his call is to determine if I can safely wait until my appointment and, if so, should he be on the alert, symptom-wise, for more serious developments. Further, what action is recommended, should they occur?

The doctor interrogates Eddie in detail. Based on his responses, the physician warns that although he doesn't want to be more committal without examining me, if I reach a point that I need immediate help between now and the time of my appointment, Eddie is to get me to the nearest hospital—immediately. He assures my already anxious husband, "You won't require an M.D. to recognize some of the things I speculate might be occurring". Concluding the phone call, he promises to provide "more definite answers after seeing her".

Eddie was understandably frightened by the conversation. Though the reason he made the call in the first place was because he suspected the potential that something serious could occur, talking to the doctor only reinforced that fear. From the moment he hung up the phone, he began watching me like a hawk. I catch him staring at me at all hours of the day and night. He panics if he calls home and I don't answer the phone, like the time I was in the bathtub. Clearly, I'm not the only one on the verge of coming unglued by this mysterious illness.

Journal Entry #3

Dear Family:

Struggling to find the right words as I contemplate how I'm going to express what I need to say to you, I can almost hear my heart crying. I feel worse than I've ever felt in my whole life, yet I have no recourse but to endure, indefinitely, until my physicians discover what is wrong with me. Meanwhile, I feel obligated to prepare you, (and myself, as well), that anything this devastating and systemic has to be very serious. And it doesn't need a name for me to assure you of that!

Lately, I'm losing sensation. Yesterday I reached to answer the phone and couldn't feel my fingers grasping the receiver. Slipping from my hand in a bungee-like jump, it fell to the floor dangling from its uncoiling cord. Additionally, I feel constant activity in my face and head, causing me to fear brain involvement and damage, with the potential for more in the future. God, I don't want any of you to know me like that!

The tears streaming down my cheeks are no match for the ones hidden from everyone but me—the ones that overflow in my heart for all of you, and for myself, because I see my role in our family, as we have known it, greatly at risk. And I have no control. I fight so hard, yet my efforts are futile, as evidenced by the severity of new symptoms that develop by the day. As much as I try to remain optimistic while this secret war rages inside my body, the impact of which is realized to its fullest extreme only by me, it is becoming next to impossible. And if one more person preaches to me that the mind can play tricks, making one think that something serious is going on when it isn't, I'm going to scream. This is not a figment of Eileen's imagination. This is real. If appropriate specialists don't take the gravity of this condition seriously—and soon—I fear it might be too late.

The longer I'm compelled to sit and wait, ever conscious of this abnormal activity inside my own body, and the associated havoc it plays, the more terror-stricken I become. I long to cuddle up with all of you and have this indescribable nightmare end. I swear, if given the opportunity, I'd be the best wife and mother in the world. I can't find the words to describe the love and tenderness I feel for all of you, but I know you understand because it's the same as that which you give me. NEVER forget that feeling—I know I won't.

With tears distorting my words to the point that my writing is approaching illegible, I'd better sign off now.

All my love,
Mom

The steaming hot bath water surrounds my body to the neck, as I lean back against the inflatable pillow unsuccessfully trying to convince myself that I really should leave this ecstasy and dress for dinner club. Instead, I rationalize that our group is notoriously late, remaining in the tub not only until the water cools but until it cools a second time after adding more hot water. Despite my reluctance to leave these soothing surroundings, the thought of seeing everyone since the long break since our last get-together motivates me.

Ironically, this group of five couples evolved from what was originally a play group. Over the years, the parents got to know and enjoy each other's company, eventually becoming the best of friends. Consequently, when our children grew to school age, we weren't ready to disband. As an alternative, we formed an adult group that rotated having dinner at each others' houses. We meet approximately five times a year. Incredulously to us, the "children" who participated in the original group are nearing college graduation. I can't think of a group I've experienced more milestones with, more memories, and sadly, more hardships. When someone is a part of your life for so many years, they experience it all.

Jen's house has never been difficult to negotiate—until tonight. Suddenly, her front stoop is higher than usual, causing me to trip on the edge I fail to clear on the way in. Her sunken dining room is more "sunken" or deeper. Ironically, her house hasn't undergone any major renovation since we were last here—the only "re-construction" occurred, inexplicably, in me.

Choosing to ignore these differences is an unrealistic option. Instead, I unsteadily engage in precautionary groping of walls, doorways and other fixed supports as I slowly work my way, as inconspicuously as possible, to the nearest chair. Tactfully, my friends divert their attention to the tempting aroma generating from the kitchen yet permeating the entire house. Part of the unwritten "mystique" of dinner club is that the gourmet, restaurant-quality dinners consistently served remain a surprise until serving time. Its become a challenge to guess the entree in advance, with most members relying on their sense of smell, though more blatant ones have been known to sneak peeks under pot lids. Tonight's is indisputably seafood, everyone unanimously agrees, anticipation undisguised in the reaction of this seafood lovers' group.

Munching an appetizer assortment of whole grain, seeded crackers, a variety of cheeses, crunchy veggies and an unfamiliar hot dip, approached hesitantly at first, and avaricely after a sample of the scrumptious blend of herbs and your-guess-is-as-good-as-mine ingredients, multiple conversations occur simultaneously. Seated, while everyone else towers above me from their standing positions more conducive to socializing from one small group conversation to the next, I feel like the little girl my father once took to his sales incentive meetings. I'd sit silently, involved contentedly in some quiet distraction I'd brought along, half listening to background conversation far too technical for a five year old to comprehend. Tonight my distraction is not something tangible, but an inexplicable internal one hidden from everyone except the complexities of my own mind.

Unlike when I was a child, I understand bits and pieces of the conversations I eavesdrop on, yet they seem so distant—like they're occurring in another room, exclusive of me. What I don't understand, and what pre-occupies me to the point of stifling interaction with the others, is the drastic, overnight transformation in the me I've known all my life. Concerted efforts on the part of my friends to include me are fruitless. The confusion and concern I read when they allow their eyes to meet mine are only matched by the bewilderment and fear I reflect back at them. Without providing any explanation for my out-of-character behavior, Eddie and I leave. Real friends don't require explanations.

chapter six

If At First You Don't Succeed...

Driving directly into the blinding glare of the intense sun, my mom squints her way toward the distant Medical Center. Though lighthearted chatter surrounds me, I'm clearly not a part of it. Lost in my own world, mentally preparing a list of symptoms to report to clinic physicians, I speculate apprehensively as to what they will find, while praying that something can be done.

After registering at the main lobby information desk, I'm given directions to the day clinic. For once my notoriously poor sense of direction does not interfere. Readily locating the area, it's obvious I'm in the right place judging from the number of people waiting to be seen. It reminds me of a hospital emergency room. This disconcerting scene forebodes the potential for a long wait, reinforcing why I don't go to walk-in hairdressers, tire repair shops or while-you-wait anythings. A sudden wave of nausea puts things into perspective, with the uncomfortable queasiness reminding me I should be grateful just to be here, no matter how long it takes to be seen.

Selecting a chair, I join the others already in various stages of medical forms completion. My aching muscles appreciatively sink into the three inch upholster padding, grateful for the absence of the uncomfortable, one-piece molded, hard plastic chairs, so popular in waiting rooms today.

Filling out the medical information sheet is time-consuming, especially the question requiring a description of my current physical problems. Even using intentionally miniscule printing, the four lines allotted for this purpose are inadequate. There are no margins left by the time I return the form to the front desk.

Back in my seat, no longer distracted with reconstructing my medical history, I'm more conscious of the patients around me. Over the periodic screech of the hospitals public address system, I hear pneumonia-like coughs and whining children, who tug at their ears with one hand while sucking the thumb of the other. There are people favoring injured limbs and one man with a puffy, red facial rash, the kind you feel awkward getting caught staring at but, to your embarrassment, your eyes keep returning to. I think I've looked away, quickly, three times already as our eyes inadvertently met. Overhearing an elderly lady tell someone she has fallen, hurting an arm, knee and ankle saddens me, particularly when I hear her cry softly as she waits to be taken to x-ray.

In the half hour that I've been sitting here, many patients whose ailments I can only speculate, have been treated and released. Just as I entertain the thought that I won't even be able to describe my symptoms in that amount of time, my name is called and I'm led to a treatment room.

Within seconds, an older, white-haired doctor enters the room shaking his head from side to side. Introducing himself as the physician in charge of the day clinic, he goes on to share the source of his consternation. Apparently the purpose of this department is to treat minor ailments. Reading down the medical form I completed earlier, he sympathetically explains, "This clinic really isn't intended for cases as complex as yours". A little embarrassed because I, myself, recognize my symptoms are more involved than those of the other patients, I defensively explain, "I was directed here by the Neurology Department". Hearing this, coupled with the fact that I have an appointment scheduled for the first available opening, he tells me he can't promise anything but that he will "do his best".

His "best" is impressive. After conducting a general physical, he does a thorough neurological exam. Drawing blood work indicated by the history I provide, he then pages the Neurology Department, who sends down a resident. The nurse who recommended the day clinic was right. It's definitely a foot in the door.

Typical of residents I've seen in the past, he is fastidiously thorough in his history taking and exam. As I provide a detailed account of the light show incident, chronologically reporting symptoms occurring since that event, he writes furiously, filling page after page of legal-sized, yellow lined paper. Absorbed in this case like a sponge in water, he avaricely soaks up whatever information I spit out.

I welcome what he intends as a momentary, thought-provoking question, but in actuality has been on my mind for days: "What do you hope to get out of this appointment?". By now, my response is automatic. I want to know why I'm having such severe and unexplained systemic symptoms and, more importantly, if the stabbing pins-and-needles sensation represents a pre-paralysis condition. I'm not expecting an answer at the moment—and I don't get one.

Instead, he continues the exam, testing mental functioning with mathematical drills such as starting at one hundred and subtracting backward by sevens. He evaluates short and long-term memory using a list of dissimilar items I'm to regurgitate back at him immediately, and once again after a fifteen minute interval of unrelated conversation. He queries me as to the name of our country's First Lady, as well as recent stories in the news. Though I respond appropriately, it occurs to me that members of the well-read, medical community use questions based on their own knowledge to determine if a patient's mentality is intact, placing some individuals at a disadvantage. I think it's important to consider that one's thinking isn't necessarily adversely affected by the mere fact that he may be politically disinterested.

Halfway through another answer, I note with empathy the resident's heavy eyelids, with only slits of white showing where his almond eyes used to be. I'm not sure if his startle reaction is in response to my voice or the gravitational alarm clock that awakens him as his head falls forward. It's a sad commentary that residents are so overworked and sleep-deprived they fall asleep on the job, even while sitting straight up in hard, uncomfortable chairs. More disturbing is the potential for disastrous mistakes, given the critical observations and decisions made in this overtired state. Indisputably, the patient suffers.

Out of necessity, I rid these concerns from my mind while he proceeds with the remainder of the neurological exam. Until now, my responses are all within normal limits. Yes, I feel the tuning fork on my ankle. I also easily identify, with my eyes closed, which direction he moves my big toe in. Distinguishing, by feel, the numbers he traces on the bottom of each foot takes more concentration, though I'm able to do so.

What I can't feel is the cold temperature of an instrument he runs along my foot, hand and the middle of my forehead. With undisguised concern, he watches me more intently as he attempts to evoke the appropriate response. His creased brow, when I repeatedly answer "No" to his "Does this feel cold?", tells me it should. As he moves the object up higher on my extremities, I panic at the realization that what I perceived as room temperature in the less proximal areas is really ice cold. This unnerving discovery makes my heart pound fast while my body breaks into a spontaneous sweat. Fearful over the potential ramifications of this unexpected revelation, my eyes fill with unspilled tears.

Something is very wrong! And finally someone else realizes it. Ironically, as desperate as I've been to find an answer, now that the time has come, I'm scared. What if it's something devastating—something I'm not ready to hear?

Eyeing the plastic bag hanging on the door, the one that says Personal Belongings, I expect him to hand it to me, as he does to any day patient he decides to admit. Instead, before my mind can conjure up any more frightening scenarios, he exits to confer with and request the opinion of his cooperating physician, the one in charge of his training.

Lost in unspoken fears that escalate out of control in my mind, I'm relegated back to the waiting room to await the neurologist. Flipping through the more-impressive-than-usual assortment of doctors' office magazines, though I should be appreciative of something more interesting than all you ever wanted to know about fly fishing but never asked, I might as well be staring at blank pages. My mind is pre-occupied with this morning's realization that I can't detect the temperature of cold metal on various areas of my body. My thoughts are obsessed with this neurological aberration. Returning the magazines behind the horizontal bars of their oak wall rack, I look up just as my aunt enters the room.

Heading toward the few remaining empty seats, we aim for two situated by themselves against a far wall. Purposely selecting them for privacy, they afford little, but it's the best we can do, considering the crowded waiting room. Sitting down before anyone takes the seats my mind already reserved for us, my anatomy molds its impression into the welcoming, soft cushion—a positive contrast to the cold, hard exam table. In response to my aunt's concerned, inquiring look, I'm not sure where to begin describing the morning's events, which I haven't, as yet, sorted out in my own mind. As a result, I ramble.

I mention the unanswered question about pre-paralysis. By the time I get to the part about the inability to detect cold, my voice is shaking and my mind is making connections I'd rather not face. But I can't help it. Trembling uncontrollably, I contemplate silently whether the loss of temperature sensation could represent further nerve damage.

Surprising myself by speaking the next thought aloud, I speculate whether physicians give patients with impending paralysis something to calm them down as the paralysis sets in—a sad commentary on the fact that minds work overtime, envisioning worst case scenarios, in the absence of a diagnosis. My aunt, whom I almost forgot was here, or that she'd overheard me lose myself to this pessimistic moment, tells me in a sad, soft voice, "Don't worry, they will give you something". But how does one prepare for such a catastrophe? And is there a sedative strong enough to make such a devastating transformation even approach tolerable? Clearly, the two hours I wait to see the neurologist provides too much dangerous time to think.

It has always been a curiosity to me that, regardless of the size crowd engaged in simultaneous conversation, people overhear comments from across the room—if they're in reference to themselves. Such is the case now. Though partially camouflaged by the elderly lady describing her accident to a relative, I'm able to discern enough bits and pieces of a nurses' conversation, taking place at a distant work station, to recognize they're talking about me. My interest understandably peaked, I strain to catch more of their dialogue. As one nurse informs the other "I'm waiting for Neurology," she laments they've been buzzed repeatedly with no response. The conversation then gravitates to the incident of onset.

As I look over, several nurses stare in my direction. Guiltily, I avert my eyes, embarrassed to be caught eavesdropping on their conversation. At the same time, I'm struck by the irony of the situation. They're talking about me, in voices loud enough to be overheard in a waiting room crowded with strangers, and I'm the one who is embarrassed!

As though the eye contact serves as a reminder that I'm still waiting, within minutes one of these indiscreetly-chatty nurses approaches, apologizing for what, by now, amounts to a three hour wait. Suggesting we grab a bite to eat at the cafeteria down the hall, she warns it closes in twenty minutes. Checking the clock on the wall, it is one minute later than the last time I looked, or two-ten. Since my stomach no longer registers hunger by rebelling with the growling language it notoriously reserved for the quietest, most embarrassing moments, I receive no internal reminder that lunchtime has come and gone. However, my aunt should eat, after all she's been patiently waiting for hours—not only for me but for my mother. Besides, I can use the distraction.

Walking toward the cafeteria, my right leg begins to go numb. It becomes weaker and heavier with each step. Grabbing the first sandwich I see, I'm unsteady and anxious to sit down. Before I do, a nurse from the day clinic locates me in the cashier's line, telling me the neurologist arrived and is waiting for me. Skipping the lunch I wasn't hungry for in the first place, I precariously follow her back, my leg threatening to collapse.

I find the neurologist spunky, bordering on hyper—but definitely down-to-earth. Her lack of a stuffy, overly professional attitude makes her comfortable to be around and immediately likable. In spite of the frightening medical possibilities weighing heavily on my mind, I feel my muscles begin to unkink, as I start to relax for the first time in hours. After delivering her commentary on how she can't believe someone with my complex history ended up in the day clinic, she verbally dissects the absent employee who made the suggestion.

Concluding the ice-breaking small talk, she switches to her professional side and takes my history. Abruptly interrupting my version of what transpired, her face takes on the intrigued expression people often do when something has occurred to them that they're not yet ready to share. Dropping her pen, she reaches for the stethoscope in her lab coat pocket, asking me to close my eyes. When I do, she places the concave interior over my left eye, asking me to open it while she listens. She repeats the same procedure on my right eye. As she does, I mention my inability to detect cold during the morning exam. Immediately dismissing the observation, she explains that the use of cold instruments is a very "non-precise, inaccurate test that doesn't amount to much". I wish I were as convinced as she.

She responds to the leg weakness by requesting a few sets of stair-stepping, "to convince yourself of your own strength". Although I pass this test, I point out, "Historically, the weakness is transient. There are times I'm afraid to stand without holding onto something for support. Even leaning over the sink to brush my teeth, my feet are often so heavy they feel like they are being swallowed up by the floor."

Convinced she really hears what I'm saying, while discouragingly aware she isn't sure what's wrong with me, I nod in agreement as she tells me she wants additional blood work. Before saying goodbye, she reassures me that her partner, the neurologist I'm scheduled to see in a few weeks, is a "cracker jack"—and if anyone can get to the bottom of this, he can.

My blood drawn, I walk out to the nurses' station questioning, in my mind, why the pre-packed overnight bag, which so many people urged me to bring, is still in my mom's trunk and going home. More importantly, why am I? Home to live with these increasingly frightening symptoms, home to endure the intolerable headaches on my own, home to worry about my uncertain future and its affect on my family. What do I have to do to convince physicians that the gravity of my symptoms requires hospitalization?

As I prepare to leave, the clinic's head physician, the one I first saw, apologizes for not providing more answers. However, he points out that by coming today, the neurologist will have the unusual advantage of blood work results by my first appointment.

Before I exit, both he and one of the nurses who have conferred with the neurologist, subsequent to her exam, express undisguised concern over the severity of my symptoms. They jot down a telephone number, instructing me to call immediately, regardless of the time of day or night, if any change in symptoms should occur. Stressing that anything can happen, the "anything" left to my imagination, the implication is that I'm better off not knowing every potential scenario. With my nerves so on end by this time, I uncharacteristically leave the statement unchallenged. But the intensity with which they deliver this ominous message makes me uneasy. As uneasiness turns to fear, their warning plays hauntingly over and over in my mind.

Eddie answers on the first ring, apprehensively anticipating my call. But after twenty-three years of marriage, there's no hiding his discouragement, even long-distance, as I relate the day's events. The momentary silence at the other end, followed by soft-spoken support, "Maybe the blood work will prove diagnostic", makes me want to take him in my arms and tell him everything will be okay—but I can't. Instead, we optimistically await my return visit. For the moment, it's all we have to cling to.

As I get into bed, the sudden shock of uncomfortably cold sheets momentarily surprises me. My startle reaction is quickly replaced by the unnerving reality that I can only feel the frigid material on my shoulders and trunk. No matter how much I try to rationalize this observation, there's no denying my lack of sensitivity to cold has progressed. It's gone beyond my hands, feet and forehead, as documented in the clinic, to much higher up my extremities.

Disturbed, I toss and turn for hours. Squinting, I struggle to read the large, orange-lit digital clock numbers. I think it says 1:30 a.m. or is that a 7? No, it can't be. Leaning closer, I verify my first guess. This latest aberrant physical revelation, coupled with an intense headache, prevents sleep. And I'm facing a dilemma. I promised to report any changes, day or night, to the clinic, yet I hesitate to disturb the doctor's sleep—something I'm not accustomed to doing. Intellectually, I realize this is a foolish and potentially risky decision, certainly physicians expect disturbed sleep, where appropriate. However, the decision is mine to make. Consequently, I opt to allow the increasing numbness to disrupt my own sleep until 7:00 a.m. when, by now terrified, I am able to justify calling at this more reasonable, though still early, hour.

Locating the switch on my bedside lamp is facilitated by Mother Nature, as she shares the first signs of dawn with laser-thin streaks of light sneaking through the sides of our still-drawn blinds. Scanning my copy of the hospital form, I locate the number I was told to call with any changes. Even turning the light on, I have difficulty deciphering the digits through my blurry vision. Is that an eight or a six? Unsure after several minutes of scrutiny, I decide to try both. This step is unnecessary, however, when my first call is answered by someone identifying the clinic. Taking my name and number, she promises to contact the physician immediately.

Replacing the phone in its cradle, I apprehensively count the minutes, waiting for the doctor's return call. My mind is swimming with unanswered questions. Are these latest symptoms serious enough to warrant immediate hospitalization? Is that what the neurologist is going to insist upon? If so, can something be done to arrest this unnerving process? Or worse, what if there's no treatment? Is this what happens when a person is becoming paralyzed? Is one of the first signs of nerve damage loss of temperature sensation? Does it progress to total loss of feeling? With each question more threatening than the last, I'm grateful when, what seems like an interminable wait for the doctor's call is, in reality, only a few minutes. Even at that, my hands tremble and my heart races as I answer the phone call I've anxiously awaited—but am almost afraid to get.

As I do, I'm unenthusiastically greeted by the neurologist, whose voice is that of undisguised grogginess. Yawning loudly into the phone, her fatigue almost sounds exaggerated. Even in my concerned state, I'm reminded of someone I know who claims she intentionally makes her voice sound overly sleepy to make people who call early feel guilty. But a doctor? Admonishing myself for foolishly reading too much into her demeanor, I try to put things in perspective. Just because I've been involuntarily awake for hours doesn't mean everyone has.

When she asks me what the problem is, I explain in a by-now shaky voice, that throughout the night I increasingly lost all sensitivity to cold, as lack of sensation rapidly creeped up my limbs from my toes to my thighs, and from my fingertips to my shoulders, in addition to continued inability to detect it on my forehead. Continuing, I report the escalating headaches and nausea, reiterating the day clinic's warning to call immediately with any changes.

As I conclude, I'm shocked speechless by her stern and abrupt reprimand for making the call. Angrily, she informs me that nothing I've described constitutes a "neurological emergency", (as if I have the knowledge to recognize one if I saw it!), and that she'd appreciate it if, in the future, I'd exercise better judgment regarding the time of day I contact physicians. Telling me to "get a grip", she hastily ends the conversation.

Hot, stinging tears of humiliation overflow my eyes and bathe my prickly-feeling cheeks. My sobbing alarms Eddie who, lying beside me, apprehensively waits to hear what the doctor advised. Assuming it must be bad news, he anxiously interrogates me. Through sputtering tears, I attempt to tell him what happened, breaking down completely at times. When I finally blurt out the gist of her message, Eddie's eyes open wide in disbelief. Taking me into his arms, he engulfs my shaking shoulders as my tears unabashedly bathe his warm chest. Through a muffled voice whispered into my hair, he thinks out loud, asking in astonishment, "How could she possibly treat you like that when you're so very desperately ill?". I ask myself the same question.

Though I experienced what, to me, are very scary symptoms for several hours longer than I should have before reporting them, my non-medically trained mind worried that the loss of sensation to cold could be a precursor to paralysis. Frightened, it occurred to me that early detection might stop this too-ominous-to-think-about process. Instead of the reassurance I desperately craved, I was given yet another reason to add to my ever-growing list of why not to trust the medical profession. Given my rapidly declining health status, and the potential for requiring extensive medical intervention, this is unfortunate.

Strictly to protect my own interests, while at the same time feeling hypocritical, I write an insincere apology to the neurologist for calling so early. Knowing she is a partner of the doctor I'm scheduled to see, and that she was furious when we ended our conversation, I compose a note attempting to soothe over the situation. My concern is that her bias could detrimentally influence her partner, whose objective opinion I desperately need.

For those of you shaking your heads at the mere thought that I could even suggest that that can happen, think again. As much as I, too, would like to believe that all physicians are objective enough to rely on their own observations, experience has taught me otherwise. In my own case, as well as those of other patients I've interviewed, doctors all-too-frequently demonstrate a biased and diagnostically detrimental demeanor toward their patients which directly correlates with the way the referring physician treated the same patient. Coincidence? I doubt it!

In my note, I explain to the neurologist that although, in her opinion, I contacted her unnecessarily, exhibiting no evidence of a "neurological crisis", as a layperson I don't know what constitutes one. Continuing, I acknowledge the rapidly-progressing lack of sensation to cold scared me and that I intentionally waited far longer than I felt comfortable doing before phoning her—specifically to call at a more respectable hour.

It embarrasses me to admit that I conclude the note by apologizing for disturbing her sleep. It is truly the least sincere line I've ever signed my name to. However, I've never been so ill in my life—ill enough to require her partner's full cooperation, void of any detrimentally pre-conceived attitudes. I'm not about to take any chances, so written apology it is.

At a much later date, I notice this note included in my medical file, which I'm asked to transport to the lab. And yes, I scrutinize every page of my medical records, taking full advantage of the phlebotomist's back-logged schedule. What concerned patient wouldn't? Attached to my note was one from the neurologist, complaining that I called her at 7:00 a.m., followed by a sarcastic comment to the affect that "this one" is going to be fun to diagnose! Doctors really need to exercise common sense before documenting negative statements about their patients, particularly with more and more patients accessing their own medical records.

As I think about this doctor's behavior, I find it appalling. How dare she chastise a patient, especially someone so very ill, for disturbing her sleep? To further include a nasty note on my chart is inexcusable. Physicians such as herself lack the dedication and commitment their patients deserve, and, in my opinion should be otherwise employed—perhaps in a profession that lends itself to the uninterrupted sleep they demand.

Devastated by blatant rejection from a physician I trusted, I lean harder than ever on my family and friends as I endure what seems like the longest two week wait on record. I rely on their company for distractions during the daytime and, frustratingly blurry crossword puzzles throughout the night. The intensity of the headaches makes sleep impossible. The abdominal cramping is so severe that silent tears dampen my pillow nightly, leaving tell-tale swollen eyelids the next day, announcing to the world a private part of me I'd rather not share. Electric-like waves of chills cover my skin in goosebumps, while pins-and-needles stab sharply into my face. My eyes ache. Insidiously, the attacks keep coming—with no end in sight.

Optimistically, I follow the nurse to the office of the physician I've heard so much about and, on reputation alone, place impeccable trust in, even though I've yet to lay eyes on him. I'm immediately impressed by this soft-spoken doctor who exudes concern, listening attentively, with reassurance that automatically puts a patient at ease. He is about my age and reminds me of a friend of ours' who graduated with Eddie. In an effort to provide as many details as possible, hoping something I say will give him a meaningful clue toward identifying this inexplicable condition, I occasionally refer to my cheat sheet of symptoms during the history-taking portion of our visit. Considering the ever-increasing number of symptoms, not only does it help with sequence but memory, as well.

At the conclusion of my description of the incessant blurry vision, dizziness, swallowing difficulty, numbness, severe headaches, pins-and-needles and other, less problematic symptoms, he conducts a neurological exam. As in the past, it is normal. At this point, prefacing his question with, "I don't know how you're going to take this", he asks, "but have you ever been sent to a psychiatrist, considering your symptoms just don't add up?"

Feeling my muscles tense and my jaw clench, my heart begins to race and my breathing becomes rapid and shallow. I want to scream as he continues, "You look too good to feel as sick as you say you do". I resist the urge, unwilling to do anything that can be misconstrued to fit into the neat little scenario he is creating regarding my sanity. Continuing, he points out that, "In cases such as yours', where no physical explanation is found for a patient's complaints, doctors suspect a psychological origin". Giving further credence to this theory, he informs me that "You don't need to see me again". He concludes by advising me to "Stop alarming your husband over what amounts to nothing", pointing out how worried he must have been to have contacted him. Once again, I swallow the urge to scream developing in my now-tight, dry, almost saliva-less throat.

Instead, I question, "Why has my eyesight remained so blurry since the lights' incident?". Shaking his head slowly from left to right, he admits he doesn't know. It is blatantly obvious from the concern lines indenting my forehead, and the tight-lipped expression on my face, as worried eyes reflect back at me from the glimpse I catch as he momentarily moves out of the way of the tiny exam room mirror, that I'm not convinced, much less reassured by his psychological explanation.

Whether my continued doubt in what impressed me as far too premature a diagnosis, downplaying the gravity of my symptoms, caused him to have second thoughts, I'll never know. However, he decides to schedule a consult appointment with an ophthalmologist and a rheumatologist at this institution. Inwardly, I'm relieved not to be released prematurely from his care—not when I feel sick enough to be dying.

As he leaves the room to afford privacy while I get dressed, I notice for the first time, a poster on the back of the door. In big letters even my compromised eyesight can't miss, it ominously warns anyone who has one or more of the following symptoms to go to the nearest hospital immediately: dizziness, severe headache, numbness, blurry vision, pins-and-needles or slurred speech. Continuing on, I'm momentarily stunned to read these are indications that a stroke may be in progress. I have every symptom listed except for slurred speech. Why isn't the neurologist making this connection? Unfortunately, my question has to be put on hold. I won't see him again until after my other appointments. But I must admit, my wheels are spinning. As a result of what I learned from the poster, I make an on-the-spot decision to put myself on a daily regimen of aspirin therapy, a known blood-thinner and stroke preventative, starting when I get home today. In a small way, this decision gives me a feeling of some control over what's going on.

Although I've had two eye exams this month, the ophthalmologist I see today, Dr. Shawn, discovers a hole in my retina, which never existed before. I question whether this could be yet another manifestation of the more-mysterious-by-the-day lights' incident, but, according to him, the two are unrelated. Instead, I'm seen by a retina specialist in his department who instructs me to come back for a follow-up appointment in six months.

My appointment with the rheumatologist proves equally uneventful, other than to say that by the time our visit concludes, I've developed a refreshing respect for him. He demonstrates admirable physician qualities: knowledge, interest and patience. His active listening skills are excellent, and he gives considerable credibility to the patient's own observations. I feel as though I'm conversing with a peer who recognizes and respects my intelligence as much as I do his. After an informative visit on both parts, we conclude that my condition appears more neurological than rheumatological, at the moment.

My neurologist disagrees. At this point, I mention that the neurologist I see locally suggested that, considering the symptoms I report, a nerve-conduction study might be appropriate. Though he opts to do one on the spot, he tells me upfront he expects it to be normal.

Before reporting the results, he shuts the door of the small testing room to provide privacy. Putting his hand on my arm, he kindly explains once again, "Your symptoms just do not add up". When I ask if the nerve conduction study came out normal, he nods his head slowly up and down, his eyes never leaving mine, as though trying to analyze my reaction. He goes on to say, "If it hadn't, we wouldn't be having this conversation". Surprisingly, it isn't egotism, but sincerity I detect when he comments, "I like to think of myself as one of the top third neurologists in the country. By obtaining my evaluation, I believe you've had a better than average neurological work-up. And everything was normal."

When I question my symptoms in relation to the stroke chart in the exam room, he dismisses that theory because I report involvement on both sides of my body. "With a stroke", he patiently explains, "these symptoms would occur only on one side." Regarding my inquiries associated with lack of appetite, dramatically altered appearance, swallowing difficulty and other related symptoms, he justifies each in his own, my-mind-is-made-up way. According to him, "Depression can materialize in the same types of complaints. For one, it can be detected in afflicted patients' appearances." The moment he says that, I recall reading in a psychology class that it often is, manifesting itself in sloppy dress and uncleanliness. Meticulous about bathing, while the clean, pleasant scent of the soap I used this morning still lingers on my skin, I look down at the crisp, freshly ironed shirt and new tan skirt I'm wearing, cognizant that I don't fit the mold he conveniently tries to squish me into.

Continuing, he explains, "Depressed people often lack an appetite and swallowing difficulty can result if one is anxious". There is no doubt in my mind where this is going. "But I have so many close friends and social contacts", I counter with. "One can be depressed and still have friends", he replies with a warm smile.

Even as he continues to rationalize each of my symptoms to fit the diagnosis he apparently already decided upon, I'm struck by the patient and kind bedside manner with which he presents it. Though undoubtedly attempting to portray the understanding therapist, I lament silently that he doesn't stick to his field because I could use a neurologist with sensitivity right now.

Getting up from the bed, I'm nauseated. My head spins as I look from side to side while trying to follow a conversation between Dr. Johnson and the technician, who just re-entered the room. As I stand, my left leg is weak and unsteady and the foot is novocaine numb. The red FIRE EXIT letters are a blur.

Before leaving, Dr. Johnson shakes my hand, telling me, "I wish I could reassure you." Given the unconvinced feeling that, by now must be written all over my face, I'm sure he realizes he can't. In a last ditch effort, he advises, "I wouldn't go out and purchase a cemetery plot, yet". Whether the comment is intended to relax me or humor me, it does neither. Instead, it reminds me of potential scenarios associated with my uncertain future—ones I'd rather not entertain at forty-four years old.

Though he feels it is unnecessary to see him again, I am too insecure to relinquish neurological observation at this point. At my insistence, he agrees to schedule a return appointment—but not for four months, while I silently question, at this rate, whether I'll be alive by then.

The ride home is nauseating. I can't look out the windows without concentrating on suppressing the urge to vomit. At the same time, I fight the tendency of my upper body to tip to the side. I'm dizzy and the spaciousness inside the car, combined with depth perception damage, makes me feel funny, like I'm in a house of mirrors looking into distortion. I feel so distant, as though the conversation I overhear in the car is really an echo from miles away.

Though my mom and aunt repeatedly try to awaken me from my trance-like demeanor and actively include me in what they are talking about, it takes concerted effort on my part to contribute, only to revert back to Never-Never Land at my very first opportunity. At the moment, it's a more natural place for me to be, though intellectually, I know it is not.

chapter seven

Fears Shared by Those I Love

Dressed in brightly-colored, large floral print luau attire, customary island wear regardless of gender, an unforgettable family vacation is depicted in the photo on my night stand. Even through blurry vision, the unmistakably elated faces that reflect back at mine cause me to reminisce longingly—to a time and place I'd rather be.

What seems like an eternity ago was, in reality, only a few years. Just thinking about it resurrects the uncontrollable exhilaration that made my heart race rapidly and my face warm with excitement, the day I told Eddie I had a "magical mystery ride" planned for just the two of us. The skepticism reflected in his squinted eyes was generated by an unexpected turn of events—our family tradition of "magical mystery rides" was his innovation—and his alone.

From the time our girls were very young, at the mere mention of that spontaneous phrase they'd come to associate with a positive outing, they, and an occasional friend or two, bolted for the car. Part of the "mystique" involved an unknown destination, including apple orchards, major league baseball games, State Fairs, ice cream parlors, carnivals, and trips to the beach, among others. It was clearly a "daddy thing" in our household that generated not only enthusiasm, but a deluge of questions extracting clues, which made a game out of trying to guess the destination in advance.

But just this once, I borrowed his idea, which I concertedly planned for during the school day, to assure it was only the two of us. Driving into our local travel agent's parking lot, Eddie's baffled expression only served to heighten my escalating-by-the-minute excitement. I felt like a little kid trying to keep a big secret, all the while bursting to tell—but I wasn't ready, yet.

Instead, in response to the "What are you crazy? We can't afford a vacation with a student starting college" thoughts I read on his mind,

I told him I'd saved "a little" from coupon shopping—"Hopefully enough for a weekend away, or something", I white-lied.

The suspicious look he had in the parking lot transformed to incredulous, as in wide-eyed astonishment he listened while I asked the travel agent to quote a price for a trip to Hawaii for four. Truthfully, I wasn't sure I'd saved enough but, if the ads I'd been following in the paper were realistic, I had to be pretty darn close. Hearing the eight day, seven night package, with only six spots left, fell within my budget, I told her to book four. In my peripheral vision, I saw Eddie's jaw drop—while at the same time he looked excited. "Are you sure you can finance this?" he'd asked, knowing even before I responded I'd never commit to a financial decision of this extent unless I could honor it. As I nodded my head up and down in response to the question, the broad smile I'd come to love claimed his face. By this time, the other agents crowded around sharing my joy in successfully surprising him.

On the way out the door, staring shrewdly through suspicious, slitted eyes, he kept asking, "But how?" to which I smiled mysteriously. As we headed home, I detailed a system of diligent coupon shopping, involving utilizing numerous stores, buy one, get one free offers, triple coupons, sale items and rebate checks. On the average, I saved between fifty and seventy percent of my weekly grocery bill. I got in the habit of going from the store to the bank, to deposit these savings, before bringing the groceries home. Though tempted to spend it many times, willpower kicked in as I reminded myself of how much I wanted to surprise my family with this trip.

When the girls asked what I was getting Eddie for Christmas, I told them a trip to Hawaii. Initially, the idea was met with green eyes. Gradually, I could tell Stacey was becoming suspicious. She kept asking what I was getting Storey. I think her calculating mind noted that the gifts I mentioned were of less value than usual. Hawaii was always a dream of hers' and I knew there was a lot of wishful thinking going on. And then, weeks before Christmas, I was sure she suspected—but I have to say, I was enjoying the game because I knew she couldn't possibly be absolutely sure until Christmas Day.

Traditionally, on Christmas Eve, with the entire extended family present, we each open one gift. We'd planned it so that Eddie's gift would be the trip, but that the girls would open something else. Eddie feigned surprise and excitement as the girls looked on expectantly, opening slippers, instead. The next morning they awoke to a tree carpeted with gifts, (other than the trip), for each of them. After everything was opened, I suggested breakfast. It took all I could do to maintain a straight face as looks of apprehension exchanged between the girls. Stacey had obviously told Storey of her suspicions, but had she guessed wrong?

Half-way through breakfast I remembered, (after having intentionally "forgotten"), that I hadn't given the girls their annual Christmas ornaments, a tradition I started when they were infants, with the intent of providing a collection of their own. Since it was the year of troll doll popularity, I purchased two of these so-ugly-that-they're-adorable creatures, dressed in hula skirts, and added ornament hangers to them. To the background music of a Hawaiian Christmas song, I presented them. Seeing the grass-skirted figurines, they immediately jumped up from the table hugging each other, as Stacey exclaimed, "I knew it, Storey. We're going to Hawaii, too!" Christmas morning or not, they immediately called their friends to tell them the news.

Considering I don't contribute a steady income, giving this gift to my family meant so much to me. I continued saving until the February departure to assure we could participate fully in our special vacation. From the aromatic fresh-flower lei greeting, to the swaying palm trees, to rainforests, extinct volcanoes, sunsets on tropical beaches, snorkeling, boat cruises, luaus, and renewal of our wedding wows in a church resounding with the music of nature—nearby tropical birds—we did it all.

Running my fingers over the smooth, shiny surface of our family vacation picture, transposed onto the cover of an island guide book/magazine, tourist souvenir from the luau, I'm grateful for the photographer's success in capturing the excitement of the unforgettable moment in a permanent keepsake. Daydreaming, I visualize myself back in that eden, carefree and side-by-side with my family, sharing fun-filled quality time. Insidiously, reality interrupts my dream, as my eyes pool at the thought that those days may be gone forever.

The ramifications of the sustained terror I experience, the longer this unnerving and unexplained physical phenomenon persists, are evident as I silently contemplate whether one progressively becomes more and more removed just before dying. My extreme change in personality and uncharacteristic lack of interaction alarms others, as well, who manifest their concern in various ways.

Relatives encourage me to "Snap out of it". Unfortunately, they have no clue that they're asking the impossible. My physician comments "I've never seen you like this". Nor have I! Friends continue their daily visits to my home. They, more than anyone, refuse to give up and allow me to escape into my own little world-the one of solitude that enticingly beckons me. And, when I do succeed in eluding their tactics to retain me as an active part of their world—a world that was once naturally mine—they fight to get me back. They're scared. I can see it in their eyes. I can read the unspoken fear on their minds. They think they're losing me. My deepest fear is that they could be right. As my condition deteriorates further, they request Eddie's phone number and that of my physician.

As much as I love them for their sustained support, I'm no longer the friend they once knew. Compared to the past, when I teased affectionately and gave of myself, I'm sad and distant. Someone I've yet to know has moved in and taken up residency in the former shell of what was once my body. I've lost my old spark and I now see the world with pessimism I never knew before. I pray my friends will know the person they lost—again someday—and that I will, too. Meanwhile, I thank God they're here for me now, as I lean heavily on them trying to get through this indescribable time.

As the month progresses, I seem to be regaining my appetite. No longer do I have to be reminded that it's mealtime. For the first time since the lights' incident, my internal hunger trigger is functioning again. I'm beginning to look more like myself in my own clothes, rather than like I'm wearing the hand-me-downs of someone several sizes bigger.

My eyes continue to bother me. I'm unable to read for any extended period of time. They tear, redden and hurt constantly. As tough as the days can be, the nights are worse. Minus any distractions, it is next to impossible to lie in our still, dark bedroom and ignore the blatant signals of distress my body transmits. From the overall pins-and-needles, to the tingling extremities, to the forceful muscle jerks, to the excruciating headaches, to the numbness, to the ever-constant dizziness, I'm a patient screaming for help from a partially hearing-impaired medical community.

Driven by fear and sheer desperation, unsure where to seek help next, I dial The Poison Control Center. Given the bizarre and, to date, unexplained symptoms overpowering my body, I momentarily wonder if I may have been exposed to some rare toxin which could account for my doctors' inability to diagnose me. At this point, I don't know whether to be elated or disappointed when, after hearing my symptoms, the agency dismissed the possibility.

Though advocating for myself is beginning to wear me down, the alternative places me at even greater risk. I'm convinced that something this serious and systemic has to be life-threatening, and I intend to share this opinion, until someone really hears me and takes what I'm saying seriously. It's my life and no one will fight for it as diligently as I will. I just pray I'm heard while I still have some fight left.

My mind is never at rest lately. It's consumed trying to think of more explicit ways to describe my symptoms. Beyond that, it works overtime considering theories of its own. The insecurity of remaining undiagnosed, while experiencing symptoms of such severity, is enough to drive a person out of their mind. Lack of cooperation from skeptical, incompassionate physicians doesn't help matters.

Lying in bed tossing and turning, I'm too pre-occupied to sleep. As my by-now, accustomed-to-the-dark eyes scan the room for what seems like the hundredth time, they focus on shadowy blobs, whose images I recall from daytime memory. Determining what the dark, motionless shapes represent is not the source of my insomnia, however. I have more immediate concerns delaying the sandman.

I'm worried about my dad. He's very ill with a pneumonia-like, upper respiratory infection that he's unsuccessfully fighting. He's been house bound for a month, which, in itself, is unlike him. Overcome with weakness and a persistent deep cough, he's been feverish and lethargic. His customarily thin frame looks frail from lack of appetite associated with this illness. Regretfully, past negative experiences with physicians leave him adamantly opposed to medical intervention.

A haunting accusation, insidiously plays over and over in my mind, whenever I look at this once energetic man that I love in a way that defies words: I'm responsible for his tenuous physical state. Ever since I was born we've been so connected. Ours' is a storybook father/daughter relationship—but such closeness has its price, especially at times like this.

Since the lights' incident, my father has been consumed with concern over me. And why not? Overnight, the daughter be loves was inexplicably transformed into someone he no longer knows. Not only does she look different, but she acts different. He doesn't understand what force was powerful enough to overcome her, dramatically modifying her mind and body, almost to the point of unrecognizable. Nobody does. The inescapable reality is that with each day, he knows me less and less. A cruel, unexplained phenomenon created a loss too painful for him to accept.

His regular calls become more frequent. I can hear the unmistakable worry in his uncertain voice. I desperately want to reassure him. I want to wake him out of this nightmare to the relieved feeling that that is all this was, but I can't. No one can. My theory is that emotional strain from the sustained stress of worrying about me weakened his immune system, leaving him vulnerable to infection, with depleted resistance to fight it off. And guilt tugs at my heartstrings as I witness his pain.

In an effort to heal him, I make a concerted attempt to camouflage mine. I tell him I'm getting better, (though I feel worse by the day). I downplay my medical visits and I make him meals, hoping to activate his non-existent appetite. As I grocery shop for him, I brace myself against the shelves of canned goods, convinced I could topple right into them. Out of necessity, I consciously avoid looking up. The vast spaciousness of the high ceilings continues to render me unsteady on my feet, while I look around wondering if the room is spinning through the eyes of other customers, as well. The obvious answer, as they continue their shopping, exhibiting none of the distress I demonstrate, scares me.

Using my shopping cart as a walker, I lean all my weight against it as I navigate the store. At my weakest stages, I wrap my armpits over the bar intended for hands, creating more stability. Though I'm self-conscious of the spectacle I make, with my legs thrust backward at a slant, I'm more concerned about falling than image. If my father ever knew my true physical state, he'd be appalled that I'm helping him. That's precisely why he won't. I'll do anything to help him get better.

Following our visit, Dr. Johnson dictated a letter to Dr. Michaels stating that although I came to him with an extensive handwritten list of symptoms, I am a woman whose "appearance is far healthier than her symptoms would suggest". He makes a point of noting that complying with MY request, he performed nerve conduction studies which came out normal. He concludes with the suggestion that I've become "phobic" as a result of the lights' episode.

Staring at my copy of the letter in sinking disbelief, I'm stricken by how slanted it is. Too confident in his own opinion, leaving little room for human error, the implication is that if he didn't find the problem, one doesn't exist. But can anyone afford to be so sure of himself where someone's life is concerned? Does he really believe he's infallible? I find it disconcerting that he documents my presentation of a list of symptoms in a negative light, when, in reality, it was intended as an effort to be thorough.

Undoubtedly, the most infuriating statement in the letter is the one in which he implies I requested the nerve conduction study. To begin with, I would have no clue that such a test was warranted, for my symptoms, if the other neurologist hadn't suggested it. I believe Dr. Johnson intentionally worded his letter in a way that would label me a hypochondriac, sitting home studying medical books looking for tests to request—and I resent this blatant under-reaction to the severity of my symptoms. When he goes on to describe me as an unemployed author, his intentions crystallize further. Authors aren't unemployed, though they may be between books. What he didn't know, or take the trouble to ask, was that I was working on this book at the time. Too bad. If he knew his actions would later be read by others, perhaps he would've treated me more compassionately. Unfortunately, as a result of a commendable reputation, his opinion, wrong as it may be in this case, is considered indisputable. His disbelief of the severity and veracity of my daily-intensifying symptoms leaves me beside myself trying to cope. I don't know where to turn, next, for help. Beyond that, I'm terrified.

The irony of the situation is mind-boggling. Desperately, I reach out to a profession dedicated to humanity, only to be treated in ways that defy that reputation. The longer this fiasco continues, the more questions I have. How can so many physicians deny such intolerable pain—or justify leaving patients' calls for help unanswered? Ignored phone calls aside, are they too confident to even consider that they, and their colleagues, may have missed a serious diagnosis, the impact of which could be life-threatening? Are medical schools inflating egos to the extent that this is the attitude that prevails? When will doctors as a group improve their listening skills, respect patients' observations and admit when a case is beyond their expertise? The questions are many but the answers are few.

Driven by fear, often exaggerated, that one's mind conjures up the longer a patient remains undiagnosed, I continue to draw my own, layperson conclusions. There's nothing a physician can tell me that could frighten me more than the possibilities I've already entertained, myself, since the onset of this living nightmare. Paralysis, brain tumors, strokes, cancer and certainly death have occupied my overactive mind. Like watching a horror show at the local cinema, these worst case scenarios unfold before my very eyes. Only this is no movie. This is my life.

The more panicky I become, the more driven I am to spend quality time with my family. The underlying incentive is so frightening, I try to will my thoughts not to even consider it. Yet, my mind repeatedly conveys the terrifying message that if I'm not diagnosed soon, I may not be here for them much longer. While I stubbornly refuse to accept this ominous prediction, on some level I must, because my actions reflect it.

As my love and appreciation for Eddie and the girls escalates daily, I reflect on a time, not so long ago, when I thought no wife or mother could love their family more. Yet terror I've never experienced before, the kind that remains the focus of your very last thought before falling asleep and gnaws away at you from the moment you wake up, has re-defined and intensified my love for them. Just the unnerving thought that I might not always be here to express it, something I took for granted until this point, compulsively drives me to make the most of each day.

But no matter how much time I spend alone with Eddie, lately, it isn't enough. I continually crave the false sense of security I get encapsulated in his protective arms. I thrive on the whispered, reassuring words uttered by his tender lips as they kiss my tears away. In my mind, I'm convinced there isn't a wife around who can love her husband as much as I love him.

Likewise, I can't do enough for my girls, I'm obsessed with making memories of "mom things" with them. I continue to prepare lunches in which I enclose comics for Storey and her friends, attend her games, make college CARE packages for Stacey, shop for special surprise "I love you gifts", bake favorite cookies, take the girls out to lunch, reserve time for quality talks, and welcome their friends in our home.

Despite pain I can't find words to adequately describe, I try to be accessible to them. Scheduling doctors' appointments for when they're not home is a concerted effort to minimize interference in their lifestyles. Unfortunately, the longer I remain undiagnosed and untreated, this goal becomes more unrealistic by the day.

Given all the insecurity associated with my current, tenuous state of health, I'm especially appreciative of the things in my world I can count on—not the least of which are the daily calls from the friend I've had since third grade. Undoubtedly the most trying time in my life, I don't know how I'd get through it without her unrelenting support.

When you've known someone since the age of eight, there aren't many people who know and understand you better. There is an indescribably comfortable feeling between you, the result of experiences only the two of you have shared. You offer one-of-a-kind insights into each others' lives based on the past. Trixie is just that type of person.

No matter how ill I feel, or how intolerable my symptoms are from day-to-day, I can count on her early evening call to lift my spirits. Reminiscent of a special quality that goes way back to when we were kids, regardless of how bleak the situation, she can always think of something to say to make me laugh. Actually, she's one of the very few people who can do so during these trying days.

I have impeccable trust in her, a feeling that solidified long ago as she encouraged me through childhood challenges of swimming underwater and pedaling precariously those first unsteady driveway lengths on a two-wheeler bike. She always was the more daring of the two of us, a characteristic I envied. It was Trixie who took this unsure, new-to-the-school third grader under her wing and quickly made me feel secure in an unfamiliar setting. Living across the street from each other encouraged the friendship beyond school hours. She brought out a side of me I never knew I had, and it was fun.

Stretched out on couches, her unfinished basement set the eerie mood as we read each volume of every series of mysteries written for pre-adolescent girls. Between books, we anxiously awaited the release of successive ones still in print. Natural choices for each other's birthday gifts were the latest editions, which we read before wrapping them, making a concerted effort not to dog-ear corners or smudge melting chocolate bars on the crisp new pages. We convinced ourselves we were our small town's only up-and-coming sleuths and we loved our self-appointed roles.

The memory of an early adventure, intended to fulfill this dream, brings a sheepish smile to my face and the expectation of retribution from my friend for daring to share it. Our imaginations running rampant, as children's often do, we were determined that one of our teachers, who happened to be tall, thin, with graying straggly hair and sharp pronounced features, was really a witch—and we decided to find out for sure.

My now-mature, adult mind can't reproduce the logic of an eleven year old, (all right, so were twelve, I was just too embarrassed to admit it), so, consequently, I can't even begin to fathom what we expected to accomplish. I can, however, recall after verifying her address in the phone book, the butterflies in my stomach as we boarded a bus to the city in which she lived. Arriving a half hour later, we had no idea where to get off and randomly selected a residential looking neighborhood. Fortunately, a nearby police officer was able to direct us to her street, which was a few miles away. So much for the stop we picked!

Within a half hour we located her street and quickly found the appropriate house number. I remember being in awe over the gorgeous, affluent stucco homes with wrought iron decorative grating over the front doors. Hers' was equally impressive to girls from a comfortable, but definitely middle class, (by comparison), neighborhood.

With mature plantings lining the slate sidewalks of this country club-adjacent road, it was easy to locate a massive tree, across the street from her home, to hide behind. In doing so, I don't know what we expected to see, but after about an hour, our teacher anti-climactically came out of the house and got in her car, and not on a broom, (contrary to what our runaway imaginations had probably anticipated, though too embarrassed to admit the absurdity even to each other), and drove off as we discreetly observed, unnoticed. Giddy just from having seen her, we were exhilarated beyond words as we headed home from our adventure.

The following Monday, when she made an unrelated comment about her neighborhood in class, Trixie and I shared a knowing look that said we were both back on her street, visualizing what she was talking about, like no other students could. If friendship really is solidified through initiation, ours' occurred on that memorable Saturday. Obviously it worked, as four decades later we still need each other. For all she's done, for all the laughs we've shared, for the tears she shed, all the way home, the summer I couldn't walk and she watched helplessly as I climbed onto the couch on all fours—I'll love her forever.

My God, what's wrong with me? I just dissolved into tears in the arms of our fourteen year old daughter. I'm supposed to be the strong one. I'm the mother. Yet, I'm so scared. And looking into Storey's sweet face just put into perspective how much I stand to lose. More importantly, how much she does.

I don't even know myself anymore. What happened to that tough exterior I show the world? How can I be so vulnerable in front of Storey? How dare I sob on her shoulders, with her little arms lovingly wrapped around me? What's wrong with this picture? I should soothingly be telling her everything is going to be all right. Instead, she repeats these words, over and over, to me. Yet, nothing about the way I look, feel or act gives credibility to what she is saying. And the tears pooling in her almond eyes tells me that, even to her, her words lack conviction.

How scared she must be! I want so badly to reassure her, but I can't until the medical profession can reassure me, and I don't mean by denying what is going on. I need specific answers to what medical phenomenon triggered such a dramatic upheaval in my world, and what, if anything, can be done to reverse it. And I need those answers now!

It's times like this that I'm amazed by the depth of Storey's maturity. Wasn't it just yesterday that she was my little girl? Yet the caring eyes that now reflect such sensitivity back at mine are far more perceptive than those of a child. Could they really be the same ones that looked at me so inquisitively, fourteen years ago, when we first met at Logan Airport?

Just five months old, our beautiful adoptive daughter, with delicate featured, porcelain, China-doll looks, arrived from Korea to make her home in America—and solidify her place in our hearts, forever. In spite of the dried, crusty tear on her flawless face, the remains of ear discomfort she experienced during landing, she was smiling with arms outstretched to us, indicating she wanted to be picked up. Little did I know, that unforgettable day, as I lovingly wrapped my arms around her for the first time, before an audience of hundreds of people witnessing my uncontrollable tears of happiness, that the day would come when I'd be in her arms. Only this time, the tears are not of joy, nor are they mine alone. As we embrace, our tears join together just as our hearts did so many years ago. Is there any wonder, when people tell me how lucky Storey is, my immediate response is I'm the lucky one? There is no doubt in my mind that she was handpicked, by God, to be a member of our family—and I thank him for it everyday.

Journal Entry #4

Dear Family:

I'm having an incredibly rough time with all of this. As I notice more and more nerve involvement and less sensitivity to cold, I'm terrified. And I've just learned about damage to the retina of my eye.

My best guess, at this point, is that I had a stroke which occurred when I saw those lights, damaging my entire nervous system. I think my physicians are having difficulty diagnosing it because it didn't show on x-ray, which, to my understanding can happen, depending on when the procedure was done in relation to the incident.

My theory lacks credibility with the medical profession because strokes generally affect only one side of the body. Unfortunately, they certainly CAN, and do, on occasion, involve both according to the homework I've done. Without ever knowing the types of symptoms which constitute a stroke, I've complained to one doctor after another regarding difficulty swallowing, numbness and headaches. Just this past week, I saw a chart which listed the warning signs of a stroke. ALL of these symptoms were on it. However, my physicians continue to insist I didn't have one. I fear they're wrong—more importantly, I fear I'm right.

With this fear comes indescribable stress I've never lived before. From day-to-day, I don't know what frightening symptom will surface next, nor can I stop this vicious cycle. As a result, my biggest concern remains all of you, the people who mean the most to me. I worry about the uncertainty of my future and your coping mechanisms. As much as I long to turn back the hands of time, to a happier and healthier point in our lives, I can't. I know you're praying as hard as I am for a resolution to this madness. Meanwhile, never forget that I love each of you more than words can convey. Indisputably, you are the best family a wife and mother could ask for.

Love,
Mom

Of the many groups of friends I'm fortunate to be a part of, there's one in particular whose surface apathy is the hardest for me to accept—probably because I feel so close to them. I say "surface apathy" because, in my heart, I know everyone of them cares. But in my desperation, knowing this intellectually is not enough; I crave demonstrable evidence. Though a few communicate their concern, one-to-one with me, when we convene as a group, it's basically small talk. A fly eavesdropping on the wall would get the impression that life is always great, with the depth of feelings beyond this superficiality never explored. As I sit there trying to focus my blurry vision on each of their faces, it occurs to me that I'm not the only one with things on my mind. The pre-occupied intensity in some of their eyes is incongruous with their ever present, social smiles. Resisting the urge to double over from the pain, I want to scream at them that we're here for each other—but not really. This is not what real friendship is about. I want to tell them I'm hurting and admit that I'm scared I'm dying. I want to share things with them that I wouldn't feel comfortable sharing with others. And I want them to really hear me—not deny my feelings. I want to cry with them but the tears begging to be released remain unshed, with the real issues camouflaged from the people I care about, as I, too, contribute to the front that life is consistently great.

At times, I get the impression they believe avoiding the topic will somehow make this horrific illness less real. Well let me assure you from firsthand experience, it doesn't! Day after day, my world revolves around intensifying pain. The tear stains causing the ink to run on so many pages of my rough draft of this manuscript serves as tangible evidence of the intolerable episodes. Some of my most descriptive writing was done in the midst of experiencing the worst events, describing them firsthand, as they unfolded. Most of my inner thoughts formulate as I lie awake in the early morning hours, robbed of sleep by the unendurable pain and consumed with thoughts revolving around my uncertain future. In desperation, I gravitate toward the friends who do remain supportive—thanking God that they're there for me as I face the intolerable physical challenges each day brings.

chapter eight

Time to Bite the Bullet

Somewhat hesitantly, I bite the bullet and enter Dr. Sheldon's waiting room. Though her reputation as a neurological diagnostician is well-respected throughout our state, I've intentionally avoided consulting her. My reluctance stems from what I hope are just rumors regarding her abrasive personality. Besides, I'm in no position to reject a neurological expert, questionable bedside manner or not.

Making an appointment was no routine procedure. My stomach in a knot, the ringing phone was interrupted midway between the second and third rings, by her staff, asking the reason for my call. Briefly describing my symptoms, I requested a consultation with the neurologist. Somewhat taken aback by her curt, "I don't know if the doctor will agree to see you", the word ATTITUDE flashed across my mind in neon, capital letters. "I'll discuss your case with her and get back to you", came the abrupt end to our conversation.

Insecure as a job applicant awaiting a decision following an interview, I tried to second guess whether I passed the telephone screening process. With new-found respect for what the unemployed go through, I sat in close proximity of the phone, willing it to ring, the whole time knowing in my heart I had so much more at risk than a job.

Immediately recognizing the familiar voice on the other end as that of the person I spoke to yesterday, I'm informed, "The doctor has agreed to see you—but only to evaluate one of your symptoms, specifically the numbness". Though it seems odd that she'd be concerned with just one aspect of what's going on, it's a start. Besides, I'm not in a position to argue, having been granted an obviously coveted spot. Silently questioning what I'd gotten myself into, she ended the conversation instructing me to bring all my medical records to the appointment.

Apprehensive as I awaited this impending visit, I also anxiously counted the five days until it arrived. It was the main topic of conversation with my friends at our breakfasts. Curled up on the couch in an afghan, which came on and off repeatedly, depending on where I was in my cycle of chills, it was encouraging to see the hope registered in my friends' eyes, and spoken in their voices, as we discussed the up-and-coming appointment. "Hang in there! This will be the doctor who can help you. I can just feel it", one comments optimistically. "Trust me, she'll take one look at you and know immediately that something's wrong. Remember, this physician is known for cracking challenging cases", supports another.

The thing that was most apparent to me, as I listened to their concerned words and read their kind faces, is how much they cared. I'm so lucky to have them. I don't know how I would have made it this far, living such an indescribable nightmare, if it weren't for their support. If I sense any regret on their parts, it is that they feel helpless. Beyond that, they miss the me they use to know—and so do I. For all our sakes, we need her back.

The part my friends don't verbalize is how scared they are. They don't have to. It's written all over their faces, reflected in their actions and, at times, misting in their eyes. I don't know if I could be as strong as they, if, God forbid, one of these friends I love changed so dramatically—though I pray I would.

No longer resembling the person they've shared so many memories with over the years, one friend alludes to the dark rings which circle what she describes as "sad eyes". Their uncharacteristic lack of sparkle accurately reflects how ill I feel. Another urges me to eat, asking with undisguised concern, "Eileen how much weight have you lost all together?". Reluctantly, I admit to the twenty-five pound drop, not counting what I've begun to gain back. Somehow, just verbalizing the figure makes it more ominous.

We discuss my personality changes openly. I appreciate the opportunity to interact with people who share their honest impressions with me—even negative ones. Their truthfulness encourages me to open up to them. They don't hesitate to point out I'm a different person, almost foreign to them, compared to the friend they once knew. I'm sad, scared and quiet all the time, which is so out-of-character for me. Left to converse among themselves, they can't help but notice my detachment. It's like my own little world is no longer a part of theirs'. That, in itself, scares them almost as much as it does me. Though I feel their gentle, (and sometimes not so gentle!), tugs to win me back, something out of my control resists. I'm convinced some to-date undiagnosed phenomenon occurred which played havoc with my circuitry. I compare it to the inside of a kaleidoscope, whose colored chips originally created one pattern, which represents the person I was until the lights' incident. The person I've become, since then, is so different, it is as though someone shook me, like a kaleidoscope and re-distributed the pieces. The components are the same but they form a totally different and unrecognizable pattern. My question is what displaced that original configuration and can anything be done to get it back?

Tonight is Open House at Storey's high school. Just the thought of this annual event conjures up hungry and tired parents, spending their customary dinner hour in obligatory long lines outside each subject area classroom. As Eddie and I approach the school, the filled to capacity parking lot, coupled with the long line of cars behind us signaling into the same driveway, warns us that this year is no exception. But we have no regrets. Standing in line is small concession to send our daughter to a school that prioritizes the self-esteem of EACH of its students to the degree this one does. Inarguably, feeling positive about themselves sets the stage for optimal learning. In retrospect, we wish Stacey had gone to this private, Catholic girls' school.

Stopping at the first table when we enter the school, we're given our daughter's report card. Stepping to the side of the crowded corridor, we quickly survey what we've come to expect from Storey: exemplary work. A subtle look of pride, meant only for each other, represents silent but effective communication between us. We're intentionally discreet because the looks between other parents vary considerably. Many are pleased, some reflect relief, others show disappointment, concern and, in one case, anger. Silently thanking God for Storey's positive performance, Eddie and I take our place in the line outside her Latin classroom.

As we do, I'm overcome with the by-now, all-too-familiar, body-wrenching chills. Looking at my bare arm, the skin is similar to that of a chicken, with raised, pencil-point sized bumps replacing what was once smooth. From my aerial perspective, countless light hairs stand up straight, towering above them. Earlier today, I experienced about two hours of the same chills, one minute on, one minute off. Starting with a tightening cramp in the center of my abdomen, and radiating to the tips of my extremities, these harmless-looking, textured bumps are accompanied by nausea. Though I can't see my face at the moment, my guess is it is pasty and chalk-like, as it was earlier. Fighting the urge to double over from the pain, while concertedly suppressing the need to vomit, I hypocritically contort my lips into a smile as our turn arrives to meet Storey's teacher. In each successive classroom, I do the same, determined to make it through the introduction. Ignoring my body's screams of pain, I'm too stubborn to blow my cover. By the end of the evening, it is a proud, but desperately ill mother, still engulfed by body-shaking chills, who heads home with her husband.

The chills continue throughout the night. Even with the heat on high on this mild, sixty-five degree evening, I'm freezing. Shivering violently, I quickly slide my body into a warm, high collared flannel nightgown. The momentary exposure of my skin to the air causes it to shrivel further. My trembling fingers struggle to steady themselves enough to fasten the buttons. With chattering teeth, the kind you'd expect jack hammer operators to have, I quickly climb between my cozy, flannel sheets. Even under a handmade quilt and two tightly-stitched afghans, I can't get warm. Unable to alleviate the chills or, more importantly, the accompanying cramps, I lie awake all night. At 7:00 a.m., after twelve consecutive hours, the chills subside.

The anxiety I feel over my first visit with the new neurologist escalates as I sit in her waiting room. Just minutes before, I handed my medical records to the receptionist. As I attempt to dilute my apprehension by conversing with the friend who drove me, my attention is drawn to the medical assistant. With my records in hand, in a loud, disapproving voice that I recognize as that of the person I spoke with over the phone, she remarks to the receptionist, "The doctor isn't going to like THIS at all". Proceeding to name four physicians I've already seen, she asks the rhetorical question, "What does she expect us to do for the her?".

Ignoring the unprofessionalism behind such a comment, I can't overlook the uneasy feeling developing in the pit of my stomach. I feel like a child who has made the decision to go on a scary ride, climbed to the top and, just as I'm about to board, looked behind me for an instant escape route, only to find a long line of prospective riders, making getaway impossible. It is with this same trepidation that I enter the neurologist's office.

Dr. Sheldon's friendly smile and warm handshake immediately reassure me. Shuffling through my medical records, she comments that I certainly have been through the mill seeing multiple specialists who performed a variety of tests and procedures. Acknowledging that I'm still having problems, "as evidenced by the fact that you're here today", she asks me to describe what's going on in my own words. I remark, "I prefer to do that. However, I'm concerned that your preliminary review of my previous medical records could influence your objectivity." Brushing my honest admission aside, she assures me, "I've been a physician long enough to diagnose based on my own observations. I certainly don't need to rely on those of others".

A major difference between her interview and those of the other neurologists is the detail she extracts regarding the lights' incident I experienced in March. She asks for minute specifics regarding what the lights looked like, whether they had any color, if I saw them with both eyes, how they presented themselves, if I could see through them and how long they lasted. My impression, as she knowingly, (and with an undisguised frown of dismay), nods her head with each detail I give, is that she suspects the answers to her questions in advance and, would prefer that I was unable to corroborate them—though not surprised when I do.

As her questions become more and more detailed, I sense her interest mounting in my case. Clearly, she doesn't buy the migraine theory, though I'm getting an eerie, foreboding feeling that she would prefer that it were migraines—and before all this is over, so would I. One thing is certain, unlike the message relayed by her staff, she is interested in far more than just numbness.

At the conclusion of the most neurological interview I've experienced to date, she buzzes her assistant and informs her that she will examine me, emphasizing the "will". Hearing this, it occurs to me that I was just screened a second time. Apparently I passed the test, my ticket to an exam with the renowned specialist. At the same time, if my answers were different, I think there is a good chance she may have sent me home. (Discussing this theory with a friend in the same medical circle, she tells me my intuition is right on the money. This particular doctor has a reputation for limiting her practice to carefully selected, challenging cases).

Unlike every unremarkable neurological exam to date, this one indicates abnormalities. For instance, the doctor notes nystagmus, an inability to follow a light without one's eyes jumping. Additionally, she is able to positionally induce dizziness, by tilting me on the exam table. Satisfied that she's seen enough, she comments, "I don't want to put you through a longer exam than necessary, considering how many you've had already".

After getting dressed, I return to her office where I find her studying my M.R.I. results. Looking up as I enter, she remarks, "In case no one has ever shown these to you, they're pictures of your brain—a pretty nice one as far as brains go". It's the impact of what she verbalizes next that sends chills down my spine and leaves me playing her words over and over again in my mind.

Looking at me intently, her eyes never leaving mine, she lowers her voice as she states, "But both you and I know something happened in this brain, don't we?". With the weight of months of serious, undiagnosed symptoms weighing on my mind, I nod my head yes, too scared to hear myself verbalize agreement—and even more frightened to face what she has to say next.

I listen at the edge of my seat, praying silently, as she explains it's her belief the problem started with the lights' incident. She asks for re-confirmation that I saw lights and then boom, snapping her fingers for emphasis, everything changed. When I respond affirmatively to that scenario, she shakes her head slowly, with a look of undisguised concern. My already-escalating anxiety soars to new heights as she goes on to say, "I wish you'd been bitten by a tic, instead".

Making a concerted effort to keep my voice from shaking, while aware that if I'm to learn anything, particularly if it is negative, I'm going to have to pry it out of her, I tenuously ask, "Is it possible that whatever has happened is affecting my central nervous system?" "Most definitely", comes the ominous but assertive reply. In her next breath, she asks, "Are you going to be able to handle this probability, mentally?". As she does, she administers short, quick taps to the side of her head with her fore-finger, as if to more graphically emphasize the mental part.

I answer her question with, "A discouraging diagnosis is preferable to none at all, the later leaving me frustrated, with no explanation as to why I feel so desperately ill". To myself I rationalize it sure beats the psychosomatic labels inaccurately assigned to me by the other neurologists.

What I don't communicate to Dr. Sheldon, after answering her question, is the unverbalized thought that enters my mind: What choice do I have but to accept that total nervous system involvement may be a reality? Even with my growing apprehension, I don't think I fully realize the gravity of the situation, or what she is trying to convey to me, let alone the unspoken future her knowing, experienced mind predicts for me. At the same time, though I've been desperately pursuing an answer to this indescribable nightmare, I'm scared and, undoubtedly, in a bit of denial.

My fears regarding an imminent and potentially disastrous prognosis are premature. She opts for further testing before committing to a specific diagnosis. Before our visit concludes, she assures me of what she later conveys to Dr. Michaels, "Beyond a doubt, something physical is going on". A S.P.E.C.T. scan, to trace blood flow within the brain, is scheduled. I'm to call for a return visit once the results have been calculated.

I leave Dr. Sheldon's office impressed. She is, in my opinion, the most knowledgeable neurologist I've consulted. Not only did she listen intently, giving credence to my recollection of the lights' incident, she repeated the sequence of events I described, asking me to confirm her understanding. Through her, I witnessed active listening at its best.

Unlike the other neurologists, she didn't undermine the systemic repercussions resulting from the initial incident, nor did she attempt to give them a psychological origin. Because I knew she believed me, I felt comfortable admitting that I electively scheduled a counseling session before seeing her. I told her it was in response to continual skepticism of my credibility, and associated half-hearted interest in treating my case. Her reaction was sincere regret that a patient with such severe, and recognizable-on-exam symptoms, was driven to this extreme. I concur.

Though my physical condition remains unchanged, I have some peace of mind knowing I'm under the care of a competent neurologist, who acknowledges something physical happened in my brain—and is prepared to treat the residual affects. I no longer feel like a salesperson, desperately trying to convince the medical field something serious occurred, requiring expedient intervention to prevent irreversible damage. Where the salesperson's incentive is commission, my potential risk is far greater: life. Thank God for today's appointment!

That night, Eddie awakens to the steady vibration of our mattress, as my left arm shimmers and shakes involuntarily. Surprisingly, I sleep through the inexplicable event, which lasts several minutes. Eddie, however, later admits he tossed and turned the entire night, worried sick about what is happening to the wife he loves—and more importantly, what's to come.

As the headaches continue, I note there are weeks they seem to peak and others where they taper off. My sleep patterns differ, depending on what cycle I'm on at any given moment. Unusual for me, when the headaches are most active, I remember every dream. Although I'm aware that everyone dreams, before the lights' incident I never recalled more than one dream a month. However, proportionate to neurological activity, there are times I remember several dreams a day, including those experienced during short, daytime naps. And they're weird!

Two days ago, I dreamed that I woke up on my stomach, paralyzed in the legs and arms—and unable to see. Eddie, who was in the bathroom, I believe tying his tie for work, was unaware of my situation. I remember calling him over to the bed and, before telling him what was wrong, I told him I loved him. In my dream, I feared that my facial muscles might become paralyzed, as well. In case this should happen, I wanted to be sure those were the last words he heard me say. I woke up shaken, it was so real.

Last night, I dreamed I was dying and everyone in my family knew it. It was a conscious, but in our minds inevitable decision. I was alone in a motel suite, (I think connected to a hospital), with Eddie. I was on some type of apparatus, I believe for breathing, that was portable, therefore leaving me ambulatory. Somehow, we knew that if I were to go off of it, I'd die within twelve hours, but I decided to, supported by my physicians. I remember preparing for the inevitable before I unhooked the machine—bath, decent underwear, and clean sheets. Eddie and I were together when I went off of it.

I started to feel the death process, or at least what I've been told one experiences. I saw Nonna, my maternal grandmother who died when I was twelve. I know we communicated but I don't remember what was said. I recall thinking how worried my family must be because they, like my doctors, knew I was doing this. I wanted to call my dad and say something comforting to him but I didn't know what I could say to take away the pain I sensed he was feeling.

Before I realize it, the twelve hours passes and I don't die. No one can figure out how this could be, after stopping my life-sustaining machine. Relieved and overjoyed, I wake up. Understandably, I'm almost afraid to go to sleep lately, not knowing what I'll dream next.

Motivated by fear and concern, Eddie accompanies me to my next appointment with Dr. Sheldon. The neurologist greets me with, "Congratulations on your first abnormal test: the S.P.E.C.T. scan".

Though some patients might find her reaction objectionable, I interpret it to convey what I think she intends, that we're finally getting somewhere. She tells me the scan clearly indicated "atypical involvement throughout the brain", which is no news to me because Dr. Michaels shared his copy of the same results days ago.

According to the radiologist's report, there are "small, scattered foci of minor hypoperfusion involving the frontal and parietal cortex, bilaterally, with more hypoperfusion in the left temporal cortex and perisylvian region. Conclusion: Abnormal study, best explained by lupus cerebritis-vasculitis, with predominant involvement on the left temporal cortex and perisylvian region".

Subsequent to the study, Dr. Michaels contacted Dr. Johnson, the neurologist I consulted at an out-of-state hospital. Reporting the S.P.E.C.T. scan results to him, the specialist immediately dismissed them, indicating the test is undependable to the point of useless, because every one comes out abnormal. As a result, his department no longer schedules them. When my primary care physician expressed regret that I underwent it needlessly, I got the distinct impression that he accepted Dr. Johnson's negative opinion of the procedure as indisputable.

I can't believe it! After a desperate and fruitless search for the cause of such bizarre symptoms, I finally have an abnormal test result and it's discredited. When I tell Dr. Sheldon that the other neurologist discounted the scan, she's livid. "What do you mean, he dismissed it?", she asks incredulously. Picking up the phone before I could answer what I'm sure was intended as a rhetorical question, she calls Dr. Michaels who regurgitates what Dr. Johnson told him about the test. Hearing this, Dr. Sheldon becomes animated. During the one-sided conversation Eddie and I are privy to, she tells him, "You just can't ignore a clearly abnormal scan such as this, particularly considering the severity of the symptoms". Referring, by name, to the radiologist who read the scan, she points out that she is an expert in her field, with considerable experience interpreting such results.

The remainder of the conversation revolves around treatment options. Collectively, they decide to try an anti-seizure medication, on an experimental basis, which Dr. Sheldon prescribes after concluding her phone conversation. I'm to begin taking it immediately.

Before leaving, I somehow manage to muster up the courage to verbalize the symptom I still find intensely embarrassing: drooling. Her reaction to my self-conscious admission is to immediately turn to Eddie and ask, "Have you observed this?", which annoys me. I'd like to believe my word is sufficient, with no corroboration needed. Eddie responds, "Although I haven't personally witnessed it, I don't for a minute doubt the veracity of what Eileen is saying". In reality, he hasn't seen me drool because it embarrasses me so much I continually wipe the corners of my mouth, irritating them to the point of resultant flaky, dry crevices—which, in my mind, is preferable to a steady stream of involuntary trickle occasionally noted in individuals twice my age.

It's demeaning to a mentally alert patient's intelligence to verify their symptoms through other family members. Yet, this is certainly not the first time I've come across it. I've seen medical report notations, specifying a symptom I related, followed by, "which her husband confirmed". This unnecessary practice diminishes the bond of trust conducive to effective doctor/patient relationships. And it works both ways. If a patient is to trust her doctor, the doctor must demonstrate that he believes what she reports, by taking her word, alone, instead of looking for confirmation from relatives.

Stopping at our local, personal friend-owned drugstore on the way home, we have the anti-seizure prescription filled. Thinking positively, I begin taking it immediately. Discouragingly, the debilitating headaches and systemic phenomenon persist more intensely than ever. By the end of the trial period, it's obvious the medication is ineffective.

Dialing Dr. Sheldon's office, I provide the update she requested, though unfortunately not the optimistic one I was hoping to give. Hearing that my condition has worsened, she administers a spinal tap and orders an E.E.G.,* (electroencephalogram)—both of which prove unrevealing. Though she is the only neurologist to recognize an event of some degree occurred in my brain, with residual systemic damage, she's at a loss for a treatment plan. Instead, she refers me to another out-of-state hospital which she highly respects. I'm given an appointment with a neurologist known for his experience with connective-tissue disease brain involvement.

Meanwhile, I lie awake every night, unable to sleep through the intense pain and incessant activity insidiously overtaking every part of my body. Involuntary muscle jerking now occurs hundreds of times throughout the day and night. Strong, forceful jolts shock my limbs, sending my appendages jumping as though a defibrillator was used. It's unnerving to have no control over such extreme movement, which occurs without warning. The thrusts are so intense, they hurt other limbs and joints, particularly my shoulder replacement site. On the rare occasions I am asleep, I'm startled awake.

In addition, I've noticed a buzzing in my right ear and on the surface of my left kneecap. The vibration on the electric-like phenomenon on the knee can be felt not only internally, but by applying a hand to the surface. The sensation is similar to that produced by the tuning forks physicians use. Curious, I ask Eddie if he can feel it, which he can, merely by lightly touching my knee.

Tears spill freely down well-traveled, familiar tracks, lubricating my cheeks from pain that continues, and intensifies, while I ask myself how long a body can withstand it. Subsisting in a world of hurt few, including many physicians can understand, those who cannot pressure me to "do more", oblivious to the fact that I'm already

* E.E.G. (Electroencephalogram). A tracing that records electrical activity of the brain.

pushing myself, far beyond conceivable limits under current physical conditions.

Now not only am I writing to my family, but to my doctors as well. I'm desperate and I don't care who knows it. In an excerpt from a letter to Dr. Michaels, I remark, "I guess I don't have to tell you how frustrating this entire situation has been. Undoubtedly, it is for you, as well. You're correct in saying I'm too much of a fighter to give in to it. However, I can't begin to tell you how much "fight" I've exercised since March to lead anything even approaching a normal lifestyle. But it's really beginning to take its toll on me. As much as I want to be reassured, it's impossible when the people who try to reassure me don't know what I have."

Armed with my previous medical records, plus a summary referral letter from Dr. Sheldon, Eddie and I head toward the distant hospital. Even compensating for rush hour traffic, we're lucky to arrive in time for my 9:00 a.m. appointment with what is normally a two and a half hour ride taking three.

Odd as this insecurity may be, undoubtedly the result of observing others encounter problems in the past, my heart is always in my mouth when a receptionist at a distant hospital scans down her computerized appointment list looking for my name. Invariably, these appointments were scheduled months in advance, often by patients living a minimum of hours away, and counting the days till arrival. Regardless, if the patient's name does not appear on that all-important, computer-dictated day sheet, he is turned away.

My anxiety magnifies as the receptionist on the other side of the glass window fails to locate my name on her second run through the list. Her assertion, "You must be mistaken about your appointment. It certainly isn't scheduled for today", causes the loosely-forming knot in the pit of my stomach to tighten into a hard fist. Countering, I'm sure of the date and time", it comes down to my word against hers'. Just as she cops an attitude, cavalierly instructing me, "Your only alternative is to re-schedule", Eddie remembers the pamphlet the hospital mailed us, with the time and date of my appointment filled in. Because the last page included a map to the hospital, he grabbed it before we left the house. Fortunately, he is able to produce written confirmation that my appointment is for 9:00 a.m., today.

When he does, the receptionist sputters with annoyance, muttering under her breath, but audibly, "This presents a problem because someone else is scheduled for the same time slot." Blaming it on Central Scheduling, she laments, "I don't know why they do this to me." Instructing us to have a seat in the waiting room, she promises to find out what's going on.

For the half hour Eddie and I sit conversing about my perspective appointment, many others are processed. Just as my patience begins to wear thin, an official-looking woman, with a laminated photo badge clipped to her lapel, approaches us. Empathizing over the "misunderstanding", she assures us, "If you can be patient, we'll fit you in today". Do we have a choice if I want to be seen? Agreeing to be squeezed in, I'm given a history form to complete, including the figure of a man, with instructions to fill in his featureless face. I see through this backdoor attempt at psychotherapy with annoyance. Nevertheless, employing techniques acquired in Psychology 101, I complete the countenance, including the all-important big smile I know they will be looking for.

An hour—and several glaring looks later—the receptionist calls us over. In an intentionally whispered tone of voice, like she is about to disclose something very secretive, she tells us she is going to go "one better" and, instead of scheduling me with the physician I was originally supposed to see, "How would I like a consult with the doctor who trained him?". I question this change because according to Dr. Sheldon, there is only one neurologist on staff experienced with connective-tissue disease cases. Consequently, my original appointment was scheduled with him. Yet the receptionist, after having had a mini tantrum over his double-booked unavailability, mysteriously produces somebody supposedly more qualified. Something doesn't add up.

Dr. McKenzie, a tall, thin, middle-aged man greets us warmly, explaining, "Your physicians from home have asked me to evaluate you in terms of a very serious manifestation of lupus: lupus cerebritis." (Ironically, the diagnosis the S.P.E.C.T. scan indicated) "It's unfortunate that the scheduling was fouled up, however, because quite honestly, compared to other staff members, I know very little about lupus", he apologetically admits. Quickly glancing at Eddie, the discouraged look as he rolls his eyes tells me that he is just as disappointed as I.

His interview and exam parallel many I've had to date, with the addition of his inquiries regarding whether my legs and feet swell. To those, I respond, "For the last ten years, I've been unable to stand for more than five to ten minutes at a time because my legs get swollen, hard and shiny. Mottled in shades of purple, they are painful and weak. I need to elevate them sporadically throughout the day, even in public places." I answer his question as to when I first noticed leg problems by explaining, "As a child, they ached so badly my grandmother massaged them daily with rubbing alcohol, to help relieve the pain". His concluding comment, "I don't think anything serious is going on", leaves us unconvinced as we head home forty-five minutes after meeting him.

chapter nine
Family Ties

As physicians continue to doubt the validity of my symptoms, my credibility with various family members diminishes, resulting in the loss of a major support system—at a time I need it most. Struggling to focus blurry vision on the distorted images of people I love, my body convulses with chills. At other times, it is infiltrated with numbness. Overcome by severe headaches, swallowing difficulty and a distant, removed feeling, I'm subjected to dissertations on how "The mind can do a lot".

Part of this is coming from their own denial. Part is influenced by the denial of others. My mother and father are beside themselves, worried about the frightening and inexplicable transformation occurring in their only daughter. No less concerned is my Aunt Rose, or Ro-Ro, as she was affectionately nicknamed years ago by her nieces and nephews who, as toddlers, found their version of her name easier to pronounce—and it stuck. Reflecting back over the loving role she has played in my life, "aunt" is an understatement for this special person who is truly another mother to me. She, like my parents, remain in constant touch, desperate for a sign of improvement—yet my body obstinately offers none.

Vulnerable as I feel, I'm having difficulty dealing with some of my brothers' reactions to what's going on. As the only sister in a family of six children, regardless of being the oldest, they spoiled me. Though I could always count on them to be there, lately I sense their support slipping away—and it scares me.

I suspect the inability, on the part of some of them, to help me deal with this undiagnosed medical condition is because they, too, are scared. We've always been so close that none of us even dares entertain the possibility, no matter how remote, that something beyond our control could jeopardize the security of that relationship. Instead, we rationalize away what we choose not to face. And I can always tell when my mom's been talking to them because she speaks differently to me, with what I know to be their words spilling from her mouth. I really can't blame her. It must be horrible to witness this insidious process, knowing there's nothing she can do to stop it. She needs support, too. And my brothers are a natural outlet for her to gravitate to.

Because each is his own person, with unique qualities individual to him alone, the way my brothers interact with me vary from one to the other. Never before have these differences been more apparent than now, with each demonstrating separate coping skills, as their sister's health declines inexplicably, right before their disbelieving eyes.

One is so sensitive, I hear his pain long-distance, with the mere mention of my tenuous health causing his voice to crack from love-generated tears. A touching letter he recently sent is a tribute to the special closeness we've always shared. Through well-chosen words that demonstrate warmth, perception and an intellect he doesn't flaunt—but that I recognize and respect—he describes what I mean to him as a sister. It brings tears to my eyes every time I re-read the tender sentiments written straight from the heart. They reflect an openness void of the embarrassment that prevents too many people from ever sharing their innermost thoughts regarding what others mean to them. His letter is the best gift he could have given me—and one I'll treasure forever.

In contrast to the brother who pours his heart out, giving me the privilege of knowing him on so many levels, another calls frequently, cheerfully conversing about anything and everything except the topic foremost on my mind—health. His denial is so strong he never even asks how I'm feeling. But I know he cares, evidenced by his repeated interrogation of other family members regarding updates. He just doesn't discuss the topic with me. On rare instances when, at my initiation, the conversation turns to health, it is brief. Invariably, he describes someone he knew with the same symptoms, now fully recovered. While I need more specifics to be convinced, I welcome his optimism—wishful thinking generated though it may be.

My eyes fill till my vision blurs even more than usual, as I conclude a phone conversation with another brother. Though I haven't seen him since the lights' incident, and the onset of associated residual symptoms, the purpose of his call is to tell me that he is too exhausted to stop by as promised earlier. Knowing him as I do, that, in itself, betrays his skepticism regarding the gravity of my situation. If he thought for one minute I was in any real danger, he'd be here.

But that's little consolation at the moment. Instead, from my mother's house fifteen minutes away, he heads home.

There's no way he can appreciate how badly I need him right now, or how hysterically I cry, as we hang up—terrified I may never see him again. Nor does he realize I rehearsed, all day, over and over in my mind, what I planned to say to him once he got here. Beside myself with disappointment, a tear trickles onto one of the wrapped packages I intended to ask him to hold onto "just in case".

Then there's the brother to whom I feel spiritually linked. Though he says little, I sense his direct connection to God. And I love him for it.

As I said, the degrees of support vary significantly among my brothers. Though intellectually I understand that this is a tough time for all of them, I'm too vulnerable right now to accept that as an excuse. I need them.

In the end, it is my youngest brother, the one I held and comforted as a child, who surprises me by reversing the roles. Like a parent who has difficulty accepting that her once totally dependent child has grown into a mature, self-sufficient adult, I, too, am guilty of seeing him as much younger than he really is. It is no kid, however, who lovingly wraps his strong arms around me, whispering tender, soothing words of comfort as I cry on his shoulder. It is with him, walking hand-in-hand on the deserted boardwalk, to the background sounds of sea gulls squawking in a dialogue all their own, that I choose to share my deepest fears. And as I do, the mature adult he's grown to be assures me, "Don't worry, Sis. No matter what, I'll be here for Eddie. You can count on me. We're as close as brothers, in fact I consider him my fifth "bro"—and always will". This sad, but meaningful moment, demonstrates the intensity of sibling bonding, and the love it encompasses, better than any definition could.

The longer I remain undiagnosed, the more I begin to notice the signs of denial emerge in my girls. As their relief intensifies with each normal scan or test result, I'm concerned that they're prematurely dismissing the possibility of anything serious. Certainly with all the testing I've had, my physicians would know if there was cause to worry by now, they assume. As logical as that reasoning sounds, why do I have this ominous foreboding that my case is the exception?

Recently Storey shared, "Mom I guess I sometimes don't think of you as sick because you attend every one of my field hockey games". With tears forging new, unmarked trails down my cheeks, I gently explain, "Honey, I'm the kind of mother who would collapse on the bleachers watching your game before I'd miss it". A disconcerting thought, for sure, in spite of my efforts to deliver it as sensitively as possible—but what happened to me is serious, leaving my future uncertain, at best—and she has a right to know this.

Stacey is more removed from the everyday manifestations of this illness, attending college five hours away. Yet, she calls regularly for a status, contradicting her opinion that she "knows" I'm going to be fine. And even long distance, she can't completely dismiss what she'd understandably prefer not to have to face. As a result, our phone conversations reflect depth and sensitivity—but most of all fear that increases by the day. Tearful good-byes, transmitted via Ma Bell, have become the norm.

The frustration and longevity associated with this case is taking its toll on everyone. And the girls are certainly not exempt. To make matters worse, I've been ill too many years of their lives. For the most part, it's the only way they know me and it's not fair to them.

The perfectionist in me tries to compensate, demanding nothing less of myself than to be an active, participative mother—far transcending the limitations of this latest incapacitating physical condition, as it intensifies insidiously by the day, threatening to control my life. Out of necessity, I cling to every ounce of strength I can muster, as I battle the unasked for challenge it presents. I'm convinced my stubborn will is what keeps me going. Still, there are times my tenacity is no match for the war raging within my body. It is during these periods, when I fail to meet my own expectations, that I know I fall short of those of my girls, as well.

Family and friends can only realistically maintain the level of energy expended during a crisis for a limited amount of time. Though my medical situation remains unimproved, I've overextended my limit. Understandably, the daily visits cut back, phone calls are less frequent and people get on with their own lives. With my daughters, the changes are subtle, but evident. Their emotions vacillate between worry, confusion and a developing skepticism, with their actions reflecting their mood at the moment.

On some days they are overly attentive, like checking on me whenever I make that frightening, gasping-for-air sound that startles me awake on a regular basis. At other times I feel as though they challenge me to prove I'm well by making more physical demands on me than their friends do on their healthy moms.

I detect unspoken envy over the fact that other mothers participate in activities I cannot. My heart aches for them seeing their disappointment, yet they will never know the effort I expend before I accept the reality that a particular activity is physically beyond me.

Sadly, the longer I remain undiagnosed, with no clinical evidence to justify limitations which increase by the day, the more I sense that even my own daughters are beginning to question the veracity of this illness. And I really can't blame them.

Instead of challenging their outward signs of denial, I elect to discontinue sharing health information with them. They need a break from the insecurity and pre-occupation the day-to-day physical manifestations encourage. Though at first they seek the unreported statuses on their own, I play down their importance, leaving them to draw their own conclusions. I think they assume what they would like to believe—that I'm getting better.

Convinced in my own mind that nothing could be further from the truth, at the same time I'm aware that they don't need the daily stress of worrying about their mother's health. Instead, I prefer they concentrate on their studies—and experience other outlets through the more carefree existence we associate with the young. Toward this end, I do my best to camouflage symptoms. Sometimes, while making Storey's school lunch, I find myself discreetly grabbing the counter, squeezing the wooden edge to keep from falling down. With a quick, nervous glance in her direction, I'm relieved to see her eating her breakfast, grateful for her innocent oblivion. The weakness passes.

Today I abruptly exit the kitchen under the pretense of getting the daily comic I put in her lunch. Instead, in the privacy of our bedroom, I squeeze my eyes closed tightly as I lower myself to the bed, doubled over from the now all-too-frequent abdominal cramping. The moment it begins to subside, I return to the kitchen with comic in hand and plastic smile attempting to hide the pain registered on my face.

Nauseated to the point of consciously suppressing the urge to vomit, I stubbornly continue to bake for Stacey's college CARE packages. When she brings roommates home for the weekend, I deserve the Academy Award for my acting job. Somehow, I manage to wash linens, change sheets and towels, prepare favorite meals and engage in personable conversations with her friends. Neither she, nor they, have reason to suspect, based on my actions, that inside I'm gravely ill—bargaining desperately with God just to stay alive. By strategically leaving the room as my symptoms necessitate, always with an invented but plausible reason, I'm able to pull it off. Though well aware that keeping my true health picture from them only encourages further denial, not all denial is negative. At the moment, I think it is a useful technique in getting them through a tough period.

Besides, sheltering symptoms from my dad was effective. His health has improved considerably.

Fortunately, throughout this entire diagnostic nightmare, I have the continuous security generated by Eddie's love and concern. Not for a minute does he doubt the validity of a physical cause. He's had a front row seat as the worst story he's ever seen unfolds—and his supportive actions reflect it.

Whether it is waking up in the middle of the night, startled to find him resting on an elbow staring intently at me in the darkness, or the frequency of his phone calls from work to check up on me, his love is reassuring—particularly at such an unsettling time. But never more so than when he wraps me in his strong but tender arms, as I cry silently into his chest. Removed from all other distraction, except the unrelenting symptoms, I find the privacy of our room safer than anywhere else these days. But not safe enough. If anything, it's a false and temporary sense of security. I know in my heart tragedy can strike here as well as anywhere else—and I'm scared.

Watching the fear registered in Eddie's intense eyes, as he soothes away my tears, I'm reminded of an article I recently read which claimed husbands of seriously ill wives do their crying in the shower...Momentarily I wonder if that's where he does his—on second thought, I never want to know.

Alarmingly, symptoms intensify. Last night Eddie was awakened by the rhythmic vibration of our bed. As my body shook inexplicably, I remained asleep, totally oblivious to the incident. For Eddie, it was impossible to ignore. Watching me closely, he detected intermittent periods during which my breathing stopped, only to resume again after seven or eight seconds. Today I awoke to penetrating, take-your-breath-away chest pain. Though I consider having the squeezing, fist-like sensation checked out at the Emergency Room, I quickly dismiss the idea. If long-term, extensive evaluation hasn't revealed a diagnosis, it's unlikely a brief visit with a random physician will.

Recently, at my doctor's suggestion, I completed a Living Will. Frighteningly, unlike my friends, who engage in more age-appropriate activities, I'm compulsively getting my affairs in order. In addition to the letters I write to my family, I initiate conversations with Eddie that force him to consider what he would do if I were not here. Though I don't think of myself as a pessimist, I'm a realist. A physically debilitating tornado ravaged throughout my body the night I saw those lights, leaving a path of destruction that worsens, insidiously, by the day. Until immediate medical intervention to disrupt what I'm convinced is a life-threatening process occurs, I feel my fears are justified.

As my situation becomes more grave, I contact my especially close friend, Denise. She and her husband, Keith, are a couple whose company Eddie and I not only enjoy but are most comfortable being in. When the four of us are together, we discuss anything and everything without repercussion. Their unpretentious personalities and nonjudgmental attitudes make them receptive friends—and the natural choice for today's important phone call.

After a sensitive and lengthy conversation updating Denise with the latest health picture, I turn the focus to Eddie. I tell her I need them to be there for him, no matter what—and that I know they will be. She doesn't want to hear what I'm saying. The idea is unthinkable to her. We've always been here for each other and she's not about to accept any thing less. I detect from the sound of her shaky voice that she's crying, but I continue anyway. Before this difficult, but essential conversation ends, we're both in tears. I hang up the phone sad, but reassured, of what I knew in my heart before making the call—that we can count on them, regardless of the uncertainty of my future.

Though psychologically relieved, the physical deterioration continues. My lower back has taken on an increasing debilitation that concerns me. For the past couple of on months I've moved arthritically as a result of it, with the decreased speed generally associated with a much older woman. Spontaneity of movement has been replaced by well-calculated ambulation. I moan loudly, whenever I try to roll over in bed, waking Eddie up repeatedly throughout the night.

More troubling is my recent incapacitation getting out of bed. I literally cannot straighten up by myself, crying in agonizing pain the entire ten minutes it takes to inch my way up the adjacent night stand, finger over finger. The worst part is maneuvering from sitting to standing, with the crying uncontrollable when I reach the position half-way in-between this next-to-impossible feat. By the time I reach the bathroom, drenched in sweat from the effort it took to straighten up and slowly amble over, I break down once again trying to get to the toilet seat which, fortunately, is the higher, handicapped version. Leaning most of my weight on the sink and towel rack, I stop repeatedly, at various levels throughout my agonizing descent, when I can no longer tolerate the intense pain. Warm tears bathe my face, no longer navigating on their own, but following the well-worn trails of those that preceded them, as I finally reach the seat.

Only after walking around for about a half hour does the pain begin to subside. Lying down re-intensifies it. The longer I'm in bed, the worse it gets. It is absolutely crippling.

One physician theorized that I might have damaged a ligament. Another, that I might be in spasm. Though I can't prove it, I suspect it is nerve involvement sustained during the lights' incident.

As symptoms increase, so does my letter writing. Through written thoughts, I channel my fears. My most recent note to Dr. Michaels includes the following excerpt: "The quality of my life is declining steadily. Awake throughout most of the night, I lie in quiet darkness contemplating the future with significant doubt that I'll have one—if this process in my head can't be stopped. I worry about losing the power to think and reason, along with my physical mobility. Most of all, I fear not being here for Eddie and the girls. I'm ready to bargain, big-time, but worry that we might be beyond that. I guess I don't have to tell you what a scary time this is for me."

Dear Family:

I'm having difficulty thinking positive thoughts, lately. But one just occurred to me: this more serious development could have happened ten years ago when I first exhibited symptoms. Instead, God gave us an entire decade to view beautiful Cape Cod sunsets together, share unforgettable vacations from Disney World to Hawaii, and develop an incredibly strong family bond. We experienced so much—more than many families, for that matter. And I still want beautiful sunsets and wonderful vacations for you. I want your every dream fulfilled. Know that this is my wish for all of you, regardless of whether or not I'm able to be a part of them. As much as the potential inability to participate in meaningful times in your lives breaks my heart, the security that you still have each other, and so much love between you, is consolation in itself. I love all of you more deeply than words can express. Take good care of yourselves—and of one another.

Love,
Mom

Dr. Sheldon is disappointed to learn of the mix-up in appointments with the out-of-state neurologist, chalking it up to a wasted trip; I, however, am more disappointed to learn that Dr. Sheldon is moving to another country to care for her ill mother—and focus on neurological research. Though she didn't come up with a treatment plan to date, I had the most faith in her eventually doing so over any specialist I saw. Unfortunately, the physician she selects to take over her practice is one I've already seen, with no success. I won't be returning to that practice.

I never despised modern medicine as much as at the moment. Or, more accurately, maybe its dependency on test results. With negative M.R.I.'s, spinal taps and E.E.G.'s, I should be ecstatic, right? WRONG! Regardless of the unremarkable tests, my search to discover why I feel worse than I've ever felt in my entire life can't end until this inexplicable situation is resolved.

I look in the mirror at the blurry reflection of eyes that belong to a different person than the one I knew. With so much excess fluid in them, they run involuntarily, leaving them red and veiny in appearance.

Excessive saliva continues to leak from one corner of my mouth. The increasing headaches and dizziness are more intense. The swallowing difficulty persists, I continue to experience pins-and-needles, tingling and numbness throughout my body.

Such severe symptoms, coupled with a lack of diagnosis and appropriate treatment plan, not to mention little, (or no), compassion from the medical community is enough to drive ANYONE out of their mind.

chapter ten

Sibling Bonding

I haven't pulled an all-nighter since the days of cramming for college exams—until tonight. Just the memory of that more carefree time in my life, when good health was something I took for granted, makes my eyes fill. How naive I was. The contrast between then, when my body performed for me without fail, and now, controlled by an undiagnosed phenomenon, resisting and overpowering my every effort to live a normal lifestyle, is depressing. Unlike in college, where I was dependent on consecutive cups of coffee to stay awake, tonight I need nothing. Pain has replaced caffeine as my stimulant.

Tonight's lack of sleep is particularly bothersome. Tomorrow we're going to my brother's in Gorham, Maine, four hours away, for a much anticipated but busy weekend. Exhausted, as the first signs of daylight coquettishly announce their presence, I regret that tomorrow is now today. With heavy eyelids, I greet morning, promising myself extra sleep in Maine.

Physically, I must be out of my mind to attempt this weekend. Emotionally, I can't afford not to. Just the thought of seeing this brother I'm so close to resurrects a tender memory from childhood, long since forgotten. Four and a half years old again, I'm lying on my three-quarter bed, (do they even make that size anymore?), in the bedroom he and I share. As the summer sun's bright rays warm my legs, I long to be outdoors at the nearby playground. But the sounds of my dad's rhythmic snoring, from the couch in the next room, tells me that's not about to happen.

I hate taking naps. Even when I don't fall asleep, I can't come out of my room until I've "done time" in my bed. I'm too old for this stuff! I can't wait until next year when I'm in school.

But at least I'm not alone. As much as little brothers can be a pain, getting into all of my things—having one beats being an only child, any day. Regardless of chicken pox, blizzards and other reasons for staying home, I always have my live-in playmate. But behind bars? This just won't do!

Besides, my brother wants out just as much as I want to free him. His by-now, speckled crib has far more milk on it, than in him. His personal reaction to our mutual boredom is to stretch the rubber nipple of his bottle as far as he can, between his teeth, and let it go, splattering milk everywhere as it snaps back. Some of the drops land in his hair, making it stiff. Others leave crusty, dry spots on his face. But the game is starting to get tiring, even to him.

Standing on my tiptoes, I'm not tall enough or strong enough to pull him up and over the rail. And I can't move it. It must be stuck. I need another plan. The excited look in his eyes, every time I try, says he knows I can do it. But how?

Staring at the bars in frustration, the rail is only attached by a few screws. Screws just like the ones my uncle taught me how to screw in and out of boards in his workshop. Maybe if I could unscrew the ones holding the rail to the crib, my brother can come out. But I need a screwdriver.

Let's see, where did my father put that little one he just bought me? I know! It's in the skinny middle drawer of the mahogany dresser in my parents' bedroom. But to get there, I have to go by the room where my father is sleeping.

Promising my brother I'll be right back, in a whispered voice that sounds far more confident than I feel, I peek out the bedroom door. Unable to see my dad, I take small steps into the hallway, edging closer to the living room as his snoring continues. Slowly, slowly, I tiptoe past the doorway. As the wooden floor creaks, I lean against the wall, hoping to take some of my weight off the noisy floor.

Reaching my parents' room as quickly as I dare, (how come the Hardy Boys and Spin and Marry make it look so easy?), I slide open the skinny drawer, inch by inch. When it is open just far enough for me to reach my hand in, I search around until I find the screwdriver. I can feel my face smile when I recognize the familiar shape in my hand.

Cautiously heading back to our bedroom carrying the small metal tool with the hard plastic, see-through yellow handle, I'm relieved to pass daddy, still sleeping, with his hands crossed on his chest, moving up and down with each breath.

At first, the screwdriver slips out of the slit before I can loosen the screw. But my next try is more successful. By the time I get to the last screw holding the side of the crib up, I can't believe how simple this is to do. "Oops! I spoke too soon." The bars are so heavy when I finally get them loose. It takes a lot of tries before I can move the unattached side far enough from the crib so my brother can climb out.

Before he does, he looks at me with bigger-than-usual, surprised eyes. I don't think he really expected me to be able to remove the crib rail. To be honest, I'm not sure I thought I could. As I look at him sitting in his cage which now looks more like the letter cee, with one side completely open, I can't believe what I've done.

Emptying all the outfits in our drawers, we play dress-up for as long as we dare, whispering the whole time. But daddy's been sleeping for quite a while and due up soon. Reluctantly we end the game before we get caught.

With my brother back in his crib, I struggle to lift the side back into place. It's so heavy, my arms shake. Before I can get it up high enough, it slips right back to where I started from. Finally, I lean it on my knee and raise it up slowly. This time it works, as I quickly match the holes and screw the screws back in. Not a moment too soon, judging from the loud yawn coming from the other room.

Regardless of our early awkwardness in experimenting with silent communication, the groundwork was laid for the uncanny ability siblings seem to develop when it comes to accurately assessing each other's non-verbal expressions. The close bond between children growing up in the same family results from a relationship only they've shared, a private world of memories, positive and negative, which form the basis of a life-long friendship. This connection, which ties their heartstrings together forever, is theirs' alone. While no one can take it away from them, others can't be a part of it, either. It is the strength of this love, which, unlike other relationships has a lifetime to develop, that causes siblings to gravitate toward one another during desperate times in their lives. If ever I needed him, it's now.

Amid waves of nausea, intensified by the moving vehicle, I initiate a discussion about how ill I look. Eddie is honest. "Although Al is aware of how sick you've been, he can't possibly be prepared for the drastic change in your appearance", he admits, with no attempt to shelter me from the undeniable truth—not that I would want him to. A major strength in our relationship is the ability to level with one another.

I've heard that a person's eyes are like a mirror reflecting their inner health. Looking at my reflection in the flipped down passenger visor, nothing could be truer. My dull, sparkless eyes look muddy. The fatigue from my sleepless night, plus the accumulation of sleep deprivation since this nightmare began, is impossible to camouflage.

I have dark circles and discoloration not only under my eyes, but in circular rings around them. Red, road map-like streaks color the whites with their thin, wavy lines.

My hair is uncharacteristically dull, brittle and listless, in contrast to its usual shine. In addition to a sporadic facial flush, nothing I do diminishes the ever-present, red blotch above my upper lip. It looks chapped, like a little child's who, on the coldest winter day has stretched his moist tongue beyond the outline of his lip, while outdoors. The result is an indistinct, non-existent lip line that blends into weather-discolored pigmentation. Meanwhile, dry, peeling skin flakes off profusely, right before my eyes. Though my sunken cheeks are the only sign of the extreme weight loss visible in this limited reflection, my entire body has diminished by several sizes.

The moment my brother sees me, one thing is certain—in his knowing eyes, eyes with forty years of experience observing me at my best and worst, I've never looked so desperately ill to him. Undisguised shock and fear reflect back at me as we approach each other, his penetrating and concerned eyes never deviating from mine. Is it my imagination or is his hug just a little more intense—a little longer—than usual? Whispering into the top of my hair, from his tall stature that towers above me, "It's good to see you, hon", I detect out-of-character seriousness in his voice. In the security of his loving embrace, my eyes pool as I look up at him, too emotional to speak, yet communicating volumes.

Intentionally re-directing my gaze, in an unsuccessful attempt to suppress the fear his worried expression elicits, I can feel the intensity of his stare boring into me. No more reassuring is the shock registered in his wife's wide-eyed reaction, which is even more transparent than his. Her hug, as she utters a concerned, "Oh, Leen", is right from the heart. Much more a sister than a sister-in-law, she is truly a friend in every sense, irregardless of fate introducing us. And like a friend, I want to comfort her. I want to tell her everything's going to be all right. But first, I need someone to tell me that.

My initial order of business, after Eddie and my brother unload our bags into the bedroom, is to address my screaming muscles with a hot bath. Predictably, they tightened during the long car ride. By now, my relatives have come to expect me to excuse myself, upon arrival, for this purpose.

The moment I submerge one foot into the warm, soothing water, whose steaming vapors enticingly beckon my frigidly cold body, I get chills. Even after a twenty minute soak, they refuse to subside. To the background sounds of laughter and friendly teasing emanating from the nearby dining room, I double over at the bathroom sink, overwhelmed with severe abdominal cramping and an intense headache.

Struggling to straighten out between waves of cramps, I finally do so by leaning most of my weight on the counter and slowly inching myself erect. As I do, even through rising, thickening fog on the steamy medicine cabinet mirror, a frightening reflection stares back at me. I feel like I don't even know this person. This can't be me!—I don't want it to be me. I must be having a nightmare. But when am I going to wake up from it?

Dressing and running a brush through my hair, I make a concerted effort to look as healthy as possible before exiting the bathroom. Wiping drool from the right corner of my mouth, I contort my lips into a plastic smile before opening the door. It's hard to smile while my teeth chatter together noisily from the intensifying chills. In an effort to be discreet, I feign fatigue as an excuse to go lie down. Even fully dressed, with an afghan and homemade quilt hugging my body, mummy-style, I shake uncontrollably. Nothing I do stops it.

When dinner is ready, it takes monumental effort to shed the cocoon of blankets and come to the table. Though too ill to even think about food, I need to be with my family. My fears have attained new heights. True, I've had sporadic chills since the onset of this illness—but never this badly. My entire body is vibrating out of my control. Self-consciousness is replaced by practicality, as I retrieve the afghan and return to the table wrapping my conspicuously trembling and chilled body in it. Still, the shaking persists. Surrounded by the concerned faces of relatives who can't seem to take their eyes off my unusual display, nothing I try to counteract it, including warm drinks, makes me less noticeable. Accurately sensing my discomfort, Al initiates a conversation about the college basketball team he coaches. I welcome the diversion of attention to something other than me. "You guys are in for a good game this weekend. We're playing our toughest opponent. They're undefeated." "What's your prediction for your team's chances?", Eddie inquires with genuine interest in this sport he loves. A smile transforms his face as he teases, "You don't have any seven foot recruits arriving in the next day or two, do you?" Good-naturedly, Al accepts the type of comerraderie their twenty-six year friendship is noted for. "We might be small, but we're quick. And we've been scouting their games" he responds, a confident, bordering on-smug, smirk I've seen before, transforming his face.

As much as I try to participate in the dinner table conversation, my heart's not in it. Something isn't right. From my own little world of detachment, their voices sound hollow and faraway, with an echo-like quality—like a conversation taking place in a tunnel, instead of all around me.

My hand shakes as I precariously bring the glass to my lips, conspicuously clinking the ice cubes. Though my brother is actively engaged in conversation, he watches my every move, intently. Eddie, on the other hand, is accustomed to seeing me this way. Well, maybe not this bad. Even in my disassociated state, I'm aware of the not-so-subtle look of concern exchanged between the two guys. Their fear magnifies mine. Excusing myself, I go lie down, desperate for some sleep before tomorrow's excursion to the mall which I promised Storey and her best friend Shelley, who, as in the past, accompanied us this weekend.

Curling up in the comfort of a downy-soft quilt, its freshly laundered aroma pleasantly invades my nostrils. My sister-in-law makes the coziest bed I've ever slept in. With all the charm of a country inn, as I close my eyes I envision our night-capped, candle-carrying ancestors climbing rickety ladders to equally comfy, feather-bedded lofts. I drift off contentedly.

The moment is short-lived, however. A forceful, involuntary jerk of an arm muscle results in a noisy thump, as my flailing, out-of-control appendage knocks the hardcover book on the bedside table to the floor. Hearing the commotion, Storey and Shelley rush into the dark bedroom to ascertain that I'm okay.

Trying to reassure them, my own monumental doubts influence my voice, which lacks conviction. Unconvinced, they remain in the room with me, worried looks reflecting maturity and life's experiences of individuals far older than the age of fifteen, transforming both faces. Though each of them has witnessed symptoms I've experienced in relation to the connective-tissue disease, including the summer I couldn't walk, the residual affects of the lights' incident are far more dramatic.

Relief flows through my veins as some of the most painful symptoms, particularly the doubling over cramps and excruciating headache, momentarily retreat, leaving me no longer the focus of my own thoughts. I welcome the release from this prison of my mind, and turn my attention to the girls sitting on the edge of the bed. As I do, I'm reminded of the contrast in appearance between them. Storey's Asian heritage is evident in her shiny, black hair, grown to halfway down her back, olive skin and almond eyes. Shelley has equally long, strawberry blonde hair, fair skin and blue eyes. Two totally different looks, representative of cultures residing worlds apart, introduced by fate and connected forever, through bonds of friendship that began at only months old. Through so many milestones of childhood—first steps, loose teeth, the Santa let-down, they've shared memories of many "firsts" together.

When Storey became a United States citizen, a local television station televised the moment. Sitting on my lap between Eddie and Stacey, wearing a tall Uncle Sam hat, waving a miniature American Flag, it was Shelly's red, white and blue smocked dress, the first of many shared outfits between the girls, that she wore.

Far more important than clothes, they've shared each other's innermost thoughts, hopes and dreams for the future. One gets the impression that they know each other well enough to fill volumes of books, which will remain forever unwritten, locked in the privacy of each of their minds, to be read only by themselves. They represent the epitome of best friends: they laugh, they share, they confide and they have fun. Maybe, on occasion, they even cry together, I can't say.

To this day, I can picture the unmistakable ache in Shelley's intense eyes as, arm around Storey, I walked her off the field in out-of-character, uncontrollable tears of pain resulting from a softball injury. Distracted from her own play, Shelley's gaze followed us to the car. Returning home much later that night to the sound of a ringing phone, it was no surprise to hear Shelley's voice anxiously seeking a status regarding the required emergency surgery.

In good times and bad, they've always been there for each other. Contentment from that thought, alone, causes my facial muscles to re-discover what it is like to smile, something I haven't done much, since this nightmare began. And it feels good.

Overcome by exhaustion, I take advantage of the reprieve in symptoms, allowing heavy eyelids to close. As Storey and Shelley leave the room, I drift off. The overwhelming peacefulness the deep sleep induces is abruptly interrupted, however.

Oh my God, I just barked! Loud, raspy and croupe-like, the choking sensation jolts me awake with suffocating urgency. Desperately gasping for air, I lunge forward, mouth wide open, in search of life-sustaining oxygen.

Momentarily disoriented, even in my panicked state, I'm confused awakening in an unfamiliar bed, amid different surroundings. As my eyes become accustomed to the darkness, I begin to emerge from my half-sleep state and recognize I'm at my brother's.

As I do, my heart pounds rapidly, unnerved by the sensation that jarred me awake. Tuning out Eddie's rapid-fire, concerned questions, my priority is getting air. I can't take the time to address his panic. In the split second it takes him to roll over to me, I inhale a deep breath.

Through disjointed phrases, separated by longer-than-usual catch-up gasps, I explain what happened. Trembling uncontrollably in his arms, my heart beats rapidly, with such force I swear it's going to thump right out of my chest cavity. Undoubtedly, he, too, can hear its intensity.

Surrounding me in the warmth and security of his tender embrace, my heart gradually slows to a normal pace, more in sync with his, which I can feel beating against my chest as we hold each other closely. Continuing to lie there in the somewhat false sense of security the moment brings, magical thinking takes over: If only the strength of the love and concern of his embrace could take away this unending nightmare. Realistically, we both know it's going to take far more than a desperate plea made at an uncertain time. But just for the moment, I pretend.

Though Eddie is silent, his restless body language tells me he is awake, tuned in to every breath I take for hours afterward. Like a child pretending he's asleep when his parents check on Christmas Eve, I sense his consciousness but respect his private pre-occupation. Whereas the child is unable to sleep because of uncontained excitement, fear is the motivator for Eddie's insomnia. In the end, his own exhaustion eventually overcomes the involuntary resistance.

Long after he falls back to sleep, I remain in his arms, mesmerized by thoughts of how he's always been there for me—and still is. Throughout this entire medical fiasco, he's been by my side, providing invaluable support. Without it, I never would've made it this far. His concerted effort to provide daily reminders before leaving for work, of up-and-coming events he knew were important to me, gave me the incentive to fight harder. The anticipation, alone, got me through some of my very worst days. I've leaned on him heavily to compensate for the void in compassion demonstrated by much of the medical community.

Reluctantly, I move from under his protective embrace, as the weight of his arm becomes too heavy against my now-returning, abdominal cramps. Even the little comforts I fall back on, to help maintain my sanity during this intolerable physical process, are, at times, inaccessible.

There's no way I'm going back to sleep. I'm terrified that the suffocating sensation will return if I do. Besides, the right side of my throat, the area that the inhuman bark seemed to generate from, hurts straight down to the center of my chest. Resigned, I lie awake for four hours before the sun finally rises.

After a hot bath, I stretch out on the couch with a crossword puzzle, passing the time until the rest of the household awakens. Too preoccupied to concentrate on the blurry clues, I take advantage of the quiet, with nothing to distract me from the activity of my own mind. As thoughts formulate from phrases, to sentences, to chapters in my head, I frantically write them down before they are replaced by others, forever forgotten. Everything goes on paper, including my most personal thoughts and fears, reflecting an uncensored honesty I hope I'll someday have the courage to publish. For now, writing provides a healthy outlet at a very uncertain time.

My creativity is put on hold while the household begins to bustle with the sounds of morning. As the sliding glass door screeches on its track, the dog decides he's been patient long enough and bolts as soon as the opening is marginally wide enough. My younger nephew, ironically the one whose appearance most resembles his dad's, as a child, brings back a long-since-forgotten memory. Pouring himself enough cereal to feed an entire family, a normal size cereal bowl is inadequate, but a family-style salad bowl does the trick. Come to think of it, isn't that the very same bowl my brother covered his lap with, many years ago, as he ate breakfast watching cartoons?

I can feel my face smile as I observe my nephew balance the oversized cereal bowl on his crisscrossed legs, while adjusting the television remote. As Superman flies across the screen, his eyes are glazed over, focused intently, allowing nothing to distract him, including the awakening voices around him. Except for the absence of a Davy Crockett raccoon skin cap that Al wore constantly, including while he slept, it's like watching a rerun of a movie I saw forty years ago. Instead, as he noisily slurps the last bit of milk, I smile at the sight of his milk moustache, realizing this is more than a nostalgic memory—it's history repeating itself.

The coffee pot perks its steady beat, permeating the house with its enticingly familiar scent, dishes clink and steam escapes from the bathroom. Competing with the sound of the noisy blow dryer, shopping plans are discussed. Feeling too ill to contribute to the conversation, I retrieve my notebook which slid off the couch, in a half-hearted effort to resume writing. But my physical condition stifles all creativity. The few unimpressive words I do manage to write are barely legible due to the squiggly lines resulting from my tremmoring grip on the pen. An unexpected touch on the leg directs my gaze from the sparsely written page to the sad, concerned eyes of my brother, who sits down next to me.

"I'm worried about you, hon", he admits in a soft-spoken, serious voice, matched only by the out-of-character fear registered in his eyes. The intensity of his scrutiny scares me. My eyes filling, I confide, "I'm worried about me, too." Our hug reflects the uncertainty we both feel.

It disturbs me to have my niece and nephews see me like this. I can tell by what they say, and more importantly, by what they don't say, that they're frightened. Their actions speak volumes. One nephew voluntarily brings me his warmest blanket, "cause that's what I use when I'm really cold". My niece can't cuddle with me enough. "Auntie Eileen—oh, never mind." "What, Amy?", I persist, my arms wrapped around her. "It's nothing. I was just going to ask if you were coming to my basketball game but I forgot—you have to stay home wrapped in blankets", she laments in a resigned voice. "Amy, why do you think I came to Maine?", I white-lie. "I wouldn't think of missing it!" Throwing her arms around my neck in a hug that says she wants me there, I pray, "Please, God, let me be able to do this". Driven by determination and indescribable love for this niece, somehow I do.

In addition to my brother's children, Storey and Shelley exhibit heightened sensitivity to the increased physical aberrations evident this weekend. I can read the fear registered in their intense faces and reflected in their kind actions. Though my adult friends swear I look different when I undergo the headaches, Shelley took me by surprise with her perception. "Eileen, you're having one of those head attacks, aren't you?", she inquired right in the middle of one. From Storey, there are more frequent hugs and "How are you doing, mom?" type questions. From both there's increased, silent scrutiny impossible to miss. Touched, I want to take them in my arms and tell them it's going to be okay. But first, someone qualified to do so has to convince me of that.

As we pile into the car on this beautiful, sunny morning, I try to suppress the growing wave of nausea by concentrating on the glistening snow and winter wonderland surrounding us. But even this spectacular, calendar-perfect scene is not enough to distract me from the sickening feeling inside.

As the salty taste that often precedes vomiting intensifies, I locate the handle of the car window, just in case. To the background music of the children singing in the back seat, I silently pray, "Please, God, not here—not now". My prayers are answered when, minutes later, we pull into the huge parking lot surrounding the shopping complex, without incident.

Dizzy and chilled, I'm grateful to unhook my seatbelt, the pressure of which exacerbates the rapidly intensifying abdominal cramps. Walking into the expansive mall, I feel like I'm going to fall over. Nothing looks right. I'm unsteady and tipsy. Insecure, I find myself leaning against walls for balance. In an effort to be discreet, I suggest that we all separate and meet back later.

Instead of shopping, I take advantage of this opportunity to covertly address my now doubling over abdominal cramps. Locating the food court, I take a seat in a specialty coffee shop, where I can wait until our group is done shopping.

While sipping a mocha coffee, I notice a candle booth in the middle of the mall. From where I'm sitting, the large, colorful globes resemble stained glass. Reminiscent of my late sixties, early seventies college days, I impulsively purchase three, one for Stacey, Storey and Shelley.

As fear of my uncertain future intensifies by the symptom, I'm morbidly driven to get my affairs in order. Making purchases for special people in my life is an unnerving extension of that terror. Even the types of gifts I select reflect my fear that this illness is life-threatening. Subconsciously, I gravitate toward purchases the recipient can keep, rather than short-lived entertainment of perishable items. Though unspoken, the message behind my motivation comes across loud and clear, defying anyone to deny it—particularly me.

Our carload is excited on the way home, discussing their day's bargains. Too absorbed in their animation to notice, it's easy for me to inconspicuously lean back into the seat, lost in my own world of pain and hurt. Once back at the house, where things are calmer, it becomes increasingly difficult to camouflage my symptoms. More attention-getting than anything are the obnoxious, body-wrenching chills that once again overtake my body.

Though Storey loves the candle, her suspicions are not aroused when I give it to her. It's not unusual for me to pick up a surprise gift for her when we're away. She just thinks of it as a "mom thing", as does Stacey.

Shelley, on the other hand, is both touched by the gift and cognizant that there is more to it than pure generosity. I can read the unspoken concern in her eyes when I give it to her, privately, while Storey showers elsewhere in the house. She's scared. She knows something serious and unexplained is happening to someone she's emotionally connected to, in this case, her best friend's mom. No matter how hard I try to put up a reassuring front, in an effort to diffuse her apprehension, I can't hold back the emotion generated by what I am convinced is a tenuous future, at best.

As a few salty droplets escape down my cheeks, defying all efforts to be convincing, I acknowledge that I haven't looked or acted like myself lately, especially this weekend. With built-up emotion too intense to camouflage any longer, the kind that originates in one's heart long before it announces itself to the world with uncontrollable tears, I try to continue, but can't. Abandoning the ineffective pretense, I throw my arms around her in a hug and tell her I love her. As she hugs me back, any further conversation is put on hold, our privacy interrupted by the sounds of approaching voices.

Before any of us realize it the weekend is over and it's time to leave. Embracing my niece and nephews, I'm haunted by the unnerving need to give them a hug that will last a lifetime—because it may have to. As nonchalantly as possible, so as not to arouse their suspicions of my real motives, that they have something to keep, forever, from their Auntie Eileen, I tell them I have a little surprise for them.

I give my two nephews polished, collector geodes and my niece a pink, glass teddy bear that I've always loved. The children are too lost in the excitement of their newly-acquired treasures to second-guess my motives. The filled eyes of my brother and sister-in-law, however, indicate they're onto me. Hugging me tightly, they whisper "Hang in there". Promising them I will, even as the words automatically flow from my lips, I silently question the reality of that vow.

Wiping the corners of my eyes, I climb into the passenger seat, taking one long, last look at their house, praying to myself, as we drive away, that I'll be back.

My next neurological appointment is a month away. Will I be alive then? And if so, in what condition? I can't believe this is happening. Hopefully others aren't experiencing the same degree of pain and severity of symptoms, not to mention associated fear, at the hands of medical ineptitude and/or yet-to-be-discovered technology. Doctors want their patients to trust them but, under the circumstances, how can I? With each new medical atrocity, my trust in physicians chips away.

Dear Stacey and Storey:

Sitting in our living room crying my eyes out, it's no surprise to discover, through the glistening droplets, a distorted 4:00 a.m. on the digital clock. By now, I'm accustomed to these middle of the night interruptions in sleep. Though the intolerable pain wakes me, it is the knowledge of the physical war raging inside of me, unrestrained, and the associated uncertain future it connotates, that keeps me awake. My mind is in overdrive. Tonight my all-consuming thoughts revolve around you. I love you girls more than life, itself—and I'm not done "mothering" you in the manner you've come to expect—yet I fear I may reach a point where that decision is no longer mine. And that possibility creates more sadness than I can find words to express.

With the neurological abnormalities I'm experiencing, there's no guarantee my faculties will remain intact. Though I pray that they do, I feel compelled to prepare for the possibility that they may not. Toward this end, I feel like I'm fighting the clock to write all that I can to you, while I am still able. But how do you write enough to last a lifetime? Trust me, it isn't easy—but believe me, I'm trying.

Let me say right from the start that I'm heartsick to see the role I've played in your lives, until now, threatened. I have so many plans, hopes and dreams for both of you—and I want to share them with you every bit as much as you want me to. Just being here for you fills my life with indescribable joy. The more I do for you, the more satisfaction I get. Yet, as my future borders on more uncertain by the day, I pray I've given you enough meaningful experiences to last a lifetime. Tormented by the potential for them to abruptly halt, it hurts so much to look at you girls, knowing there's nothing I can do to change things. But, like dad said, "I certainly didn't choose this from some menu".

Believe me, I've tried bargaining. I'm willing to give up more than you know, just to be a part of your lives. I suppose if our lives together weren't so special, I wouldn't feel this way, at least not to this extent. But they are. We share so much in friendship and family times. Never forget those times. We've established traditions which, if I'm unable to continue carrying out, you and dad can. I want you to do this girls. It's important—for you, for dad; and for me.

In conclusion, I'll share with you what I told dad. I wish I could bottle my love for you to store so you could open it whenever you need it. Instead, all I can say is regardless of how this disease makes me look or act, deep inside of me, at some level, is an undying love for both of you. NEVER forget that. It breaks my heart to be in this position—and breaks it even more that you and dad are the direct recipients of the heartache it causes.

Love,
Mom

In addition to current symptoms intensifying over the next week, Dr. Michaels comments that I'm slurring my speech, an observation I don't hear on my own. Ironically, it was the only symptom listed on the stroke chart that I didn't have. Regardless, I'm far more self-conscious of the uncontrollable, sporadic drooling that recently began. I feel the warm rush of embarrassment as I admit this symptom to my doctor. Minutes later, a flushed, sunburn-like face stares back at me from the passenger visor mirror, residual evidence of my discomfort in sharing such an unfeminine, though involuntary, characteristic.

In the privacy of my nighttime insomnia, the tears flow freely. I can't stand this intolerable deep, penetrating head pain much longer. My unsuccessful attempts to fight it are wearing me down, both physically and emotionally. I'm desperate for a diagnosis and treatment—more desperate than the neurologists I've seen can even begin to fathom. In spite of incessant efforts on my part to convey this critical message, they close-mindedly choose not to hear or accept it. I don't know what else I can say or do to convince them of how gravely ill I really am.

Currently, my doctors' appointments are about thirty days apart. That means for the whole month in between I'm expected to cope, independently, with whatever is rampaging my body, and insidiously attacking my brain. I then return to my physician to report what's going on, only to be released for another month—alone to stifle sobs from pain so intense I can't sleep nights, to contend with body-wrenching chills that vibrate me involuntarily, to lie partially immobile unable to rotate at the waist due to indescribable spinal pain, to slur my speech, to drool, to fight the urge to vomit from intense nausea, to ambulate only with considerable difficulty, to lose urine and to unsuccessfully try to deny to myself inescapable numbness throughout my body. Though surrounded by others, I live alone in a private world of horrific pain and terror few can appreciate. It's a world I've involuntarily come to know, not a world I've chosen to know—and I refuse to accept it.

Poor as my timing may be, I've lost respect for the medical community, particularly those physicians who adamantly refuse to consider more aggressive treatment intervention. I find it appalling that they dismiss the suggestion of hospitalization, turn deaf ears on my desperate pleas for help, physically throw up their hands in resignation, ignore my calls and minimize my symptoms. Even taking into consideration that insurance companies hold them more accountable than ever for exorbitant medical expenses, does that justify allowing someone with a potentially life-threatening illness to walk the streets?

I resent the amount of effort required, on my part, to research my own diagnosis at a time when I'm so physically depleted. But something serious is going on and I intend to get to the bottom of it, one way or another. Out of desperation for an answer, and, more importantly, the associated relief I anticipate appropriate treatment will bring, I've contacted state representatives in an effort to expedite appointments with specialists, written countless letters to my physicians providing updated statuses, researched and contacted medical institutions throughout the United States and basically pursued every avenue I can think of to get help. To date, my exhausting efforts have amounted to an exercise in futility. But quitting is not an option. I'm convinced my persistence may save, or prolong my life—an incentive to powerful to ignore.

Journal Entry #5

Dear Family:

There are no words in my vocabulary that do justice to the fear I feel. It seems inhumane to helplessly have to experience these insidious sensations multiply and climb throughout my body, void of any control. It's enough to drive me out of my mind!

More importantly, NONE of you deserves this. I don't want you to see me like this, especially as sensations increase in my head, the long-term results of which I can't, or choose not to predict. I only want you to know the wife and mother I've been to this point—active and thinking. I'm having such a hard time with this. It's eating away at me. I feel like I'm living the never-ending nightmare. God, I wish it were a nightmare—one that I could wake up from, magically transformed back to the other me we once knew.

It's incomprehensible to me that this could happen to our family. Yet, the realities of its ramifications defy my own denial, stubborn as it is. While I pray that the quality time we've shared is enough to give us strength now, I know that no one, or no event, can take away the memories I'm asking you to keep in your hearts forever. I love you guys so much it hurts. You mean the world to me.

Love,
Mom

Scared, I call the neurologist's office to report a reality I can no longer escape: I'm sicker by the day—and I don't feel secure waiting three more months until my next appointment to tell him that! Days later, he returns my call.

With intentional tact intended to spare him from admitting an initial diagnostic error, yet still address a theory heavy on my mind, I inquire, "Is this starting to sound like it may have been a stroke, after all?" His undisguised exasperation, as he deeply inhales, is clearly audible via Ma Bell, followed by an annoyed, exaggerated loud sigh—the kind people use just before saying something others usually don't want to hear. His dripping with sarcasm retort, "I don't know what other words to use to convince you, once and for all, that you didn't have a stroke", makes no attempt at tact. As he says it, I don't know, either, because I think he's wrong. And in my mind, questioning the infallibility of his diagnosis is long overdue. His conversation-ending question, "Why do you want a stroke so badly?", tells me he just doesn't get it. I want nothing of the sort! On the other hand, there is no denying that the sudden onset of inexplicable, extreme central nervous system symptoms make me suspicious. But why the negative C.A.T. scan? It just doesn't add up. For my sake, I hope it does soon. I'm reaching the end of my rope.

"Hello. May I speak to Eileen Radziunas"?, the caller requests as I pick up the phone on its third ring. "This is she", I respond. "Terrific. I wasn't sure I had the right number", an enthusiastic female voice continues. "I'm calling to see if you'd agree to do a book signing at a golf tournament to benefit The Lupus Foundation." "I'd love to", I respond automatically, offering to donate sales to the charity earmarked for disease research. Excited with my affirmative response, before ending the conversation this pleasant woman, subsequently-turned-friend, promises to send directions to the country club, located about an hour from our home.

Honored to be asked, I'm exhilarated as I return the phone to its cradle. I love doing book signings, author luncheons and talks associated with "Lupus: My Search for a Diagnosis". Besides, I can use a positive distraction from my recent symptoms. Coincidentally, Eddie has that day off. Out of consideration, we are both invited to the complimentary dinner included on the agenda, eliminating the need for me to find a ride. It sounds like a fun day dedicated to a good cause.

Selection of an outfit takes trial and error as I dress for the benefit. Some of my clothes hang unflatteringly off my frame in contrast to when I purchased them. From another perspective, clothes that haven't fit in years, do. Actually, I end up choosing a particularly feminine, one-size-fits-all gauze skirt of Storey's. The pretty floral print matches especially well with the ecru top I select. Adding a unique, carved wooden animal necklace I purchased in Hawaii, I'm pleased with the way the entire outfit comes together, momentarily reflecting on the added benefit of having daughters—sharing clothes.

Since the days I first learned I had lupus, I became proficient at hiding my pain from others. As much as possible, I wanted my family to see me as able-bodied as any other wife and mother. With practice, it became automatic. I've given talks through intense muscle and joint pain, baked cookies when my arms were so weak I could hardly stir the stiff batter and smiled instead of allowing the tears to flow as my aching body watched softball games from hard, metal bleachers.

If ever I needed this "skill", it was today. At one point, publicity pictures were taken with Eddie and I sitting in a golf cart. Somehow, in spite of excruciating head pain and a strong urge to vomit, I gave the photographer a big smile. Looking at the picture at a later date, only I see the deception. While my lips smile, my eyes register intense pain.

By the end of the day, I'm exhausted but satisfied with the way it went. The Foundation did well—and I felt like an integral part of their success. "Please, God", I pray that night, "let me get better so I can continuè to function at the active level I've enjoyed in the past."

It's now two months since my neurological appointment with Dr. Johnson. Out of necessity, I suck lemon drops incessantly in a futile effort to counteract increasing swallowing difficulty. As my condition, in general, worsens, I don't see how I can wait another two months until my next appointment. Awakening out of my sleep again tonight, to the disconcerting cold, damp reminder of another urinary incontinence episode, I know I can't.

In an update letter I address to the neurologist, I describe changes in symptoms since we last spoke, particularly noting the sudden and alarming inability to maneuver myself out of bed for an entire week, due to what feels like nerve involvement in my lower back. I conclude by advising him that at my last appointment with Dr. Michaels, he mentioned that I was slurring my speech.

Apparently Dr. Johnson doesn't share my concern, as evidenced by the fact that it takes him a month to respond to my letter. When he does, it is to inform me "I feel that a return visit to see me will be unlikely to change my impression as we had previously discussed. As you may recall, a follow-up appointment with me was based on your request following our last meeting". Reading his letter in silent disbelief, I wonder how much more has to go wrong with one body for this great guru to be impressed. The mounting bitterness in me speculates how long he would tolerate, without explanation, the warm, uncomfortable trickling flow of urinary incontinence before demanding help, not to mention the other horrendous symptoms.

As far as I'm concerned, my association with him has ended. He may have an excellent reputation but you can't prove it by the way he's handled my case. I have no intention of remaining his patient. If a significant and sudden change in vision, sensory abnormalities, excruciating headaches, swallowing difficulty and urinary incontinence are not enough to make him re-think his original assessment, I don't plan to stick around to see what will. He strikes me as a physician who is a little too sure of his opinion to be dealing with patients' lives. Everyone, even the most brilliant technicians, are capable of making a mistake. A sign of maturity is the ability to acknowledge errors in judgment and move on. Regardless of what symptoms develop in the future, I think his denial is so intense he will remain convinced that nothing is physically wrong with me. It's clearly time to move on.

Being repeatedly rejected by physicians is esteem-depleting. Many people associate rejection with having done something wrong. Though intellectually I know this, as my condition declines, I, too, resort to second guessing myself, trying to determine if there's more I can do to facilitate diagnosis. Yet, for the life of me, I can't think of what.

Lying in the peaceful darkness of our bedroom that night, barely enduring the most intense headache I've ever experienced, the tears pool in my eyes. Eddie must sense something is wrong as he sleepily surrounds me in his strong arms, while against the warmth and security of his body I dissolve into tears. Crying hysterically, the words I sputter with my face buried in his chest are virtually incoherent. What I do manage to get out, "I feel so sick I fear I could die right before my disbelieving doctors' eyes", indicates to Eddie and I that clearly, I need help—NOW!

My fear is that I'm running out of options. At a time when I feel sicker than words can describe, one neurologist after another looks at me as though I have three heads when I say I'm ill. Unfortunately, I've been this route before. When a patient's symptoms don't fall into a specific diagnostic category, there are doctors who automatically assume a psychosomatic origin. This often premature and inaccurate decision plays havoc with the patient involved, both physically and emotionally. No matter how sane at the onset, the patient will have all they can do to maintain that sanity while experiencing severe, and real symptoms, that fall on deaf ears of close-minded physicians.

With no defense otherwise, the grim reality is that the only recourse a patient has toward overcoming these attitudes, is to play the game. To get physicians to reconsider their stance, the psychosomatic theory must first be disproved by someone qualified to make such an evaluation. Consequently, I again contact a therapist on my own. With mixed feelings, I open the door to his office.

While this kind, personable man listens intently as I detail my situation, my initial hesitation subsides. His easy-to-talk-to demeanor encourages me to open up. Specifically, I emphasize how much I love my family, and living in general, I desperately try to convey their need for me. Continuing, I refer to unfulfilled personal goals I've set for myself, concluding, "I'm just not ready to die!". When he asks how imminent I feel that morbid probability is, I respond, "Very, unless someone in the medical field recognizes the danger I'm in and successfully treats the problem". I answer his question regarding whether I feel my situation is hopeless by assuring him, "I choose to believe it is not, with appropriate and immediate intervention".

I deny his sentiments that if I have something life-threatening I will have to learn to accept it. NEVER! I'm a born fighter who has overcome too much in the past ten years to give up now. That just isn't in my realm of possibility.

As I write these words, I find myself reflecting on how many other individuals, fighting their own various and serious physical conditions, have felt these same feelings, demonstrated the same degree of fight, (possibly in some cases, more), and lost their battles. My silent reverie is interrupted with my verbal conviction that, "I'm just not ready to desert a husband and two daughters I love more than life, itself". Beyond that, I'm not content to leave this world without giving more of myself, first. As the psychologist attempts to assure me that families learn to adapt to losses and do fine, I feel like the recipient of a sales pitch for a product I don't want. Though I hear what he has to say, my heart isn't in it.

Our visit concludes with no follow-up appointment scheduled. Instead, we jointly agree that my symptoms warrant seeing another medical specialist for an impartial evaluation. To assure objectivity, he advises that I don't provide the new physician with past records until after his initial assessment. We agree that if this physician concludes nothing physical is going on, I will schedule a return visit with the psychologist. Meanwhile, cognizant of the stress generated by the unresolved and serious symptoms occurring since the lights episode, he assures me his schedule is flexible enough to work me in if I ever need to talk. With the security of that statement, we part.

"What happened to your arm?", a local proprietor asks with undisguised concern. "I had surgery", I respond noncommittally. "And look at you, out and about instead of at home recovering", she marvels and admonishes at the same time. "Actually, the operation was six months ago", I share. "And you're still in a wrist splint and sling!", she observes incredulously. "I assumed it was carpal tunnel, but not for that long. You know, it's strange but for as many times as you've been in here since, I never noticed it." Good job camouflaging it with clothing, Eileen, I commend myself in silent satisfaction.

To me, symptomatic stop-gap surgery is so commonplace in treating the inflammation associated with connective-tissue disease, it didn't occur to me to justify space in these pages mentioning it—until now, in describing the reaction of someone else. But the penetrating concern in eyes that focus on mine weakens me into spontaneous honesty, surprising myself. "I have lupus. The surgery was the result of a complication of the disease", I share. Upon hearing this, she immediately averts her gaze downward. When she again makes eye contact, after what appears a deliberate interruption, I look into glassy pools of pain only someone with firsthand experience could know. "I was very close to a lupus patient", she utters softly. "She died", I state the obvious. The sad, but affirmative nod comes as no surprise. Suddenly, my interest is uncontained. "Do you mind sharing the specific complication that took her life?", I inquire cautiously, aware that statistically, my guess as to the patient's gender was a logical and accurate assumption. Solemnly, she informs me, "She was having multiple strokes. Though her pain was horrendous, she was repeatedly labeled a hypochondriac. The final stroke was too intense to survive regardless of her fighting spirit. On autopsy, numerous others were discovered. I'll pray that's not your fate", she promises genuinely. Trying not to let my expression show how unnerved this information left me, in an effort to spare the feelings of this obviously sensitive person, I smile, responding, "Thanks", and exit soon after—more shaken from within, by this latest revelation, than she could ever know.

chapter eleven
Not More Doctors!

It's with a tightening knot of trepidation, spewing cramps throughout my stomach, that Eddie and I drive to the cardiologist's. Dr. Michaels' referral results from the chest pain associated with the barking incident. Undoubtedly, the nervousness eating away at me reflects discouragement of months of negative and disappointing visits with various specialists, while my unspoken thoughts prepare for the reality that I could be setting myself up for, yet, another one.

Counteracting this uncomfortable feeling in my gut are twinges of optimism, regardless of my body's mute, but effective, way of warning me that this could be a mistake. Despite remaining undiagnosed for so long, I've got to believe somewhere there is a physician who can make this nightmare end. To think otherwise would rob me of my sanity.

The cardiologist's entrance interrupts the by-now, all-too-familiar words of the silent, unanswered prayer that consumes my thoughts prior to meeting each new specialist. Dr. Cohen immediately impresses me with the credibility he lends my personal account of the historical background of this illness. In unmistakable ways, he conveys what I have to say is important to him. For starters, he explains, "Although I have an introductory letter from Dr. Michaels, I'd prefer to hear what's occurring in your own words". Complying with this esteem-stroking request, I describe the lights' incident and detail subsequent events. Meticulously taking notes, he listens without interruption, except for occasional sequence clarification immediately followed by encouragement to resume. He is quick to nod agreement to observations I make, periodically complimenting both the historical value of my account, as well as the intellect reflected by it. This is a far cry from the doctors who looked at me like I had two heads when I described some of my bizarre, but none-the-less real symptoms. Not once does he give the impression that he is enamored with the fact that he is a physician, or that his ego is so inflated he's too above me to converse at my level. If anything, he conveys just the opposite. The description I give is clearly an essential piece of his evaluation.

During the physical exam, he devotes particular emphasis to pulses throughout the body. With his stethoscope he listens not only to my chest but to the entire abdominal region. Hesitating for much longer in one area around the navel, long enough for the initially cold stethoscope to warm up to room temperature, he asks, "Does this hurt?". As he does, I can feel my stomach muscles knot in anxiety, while I reluctantly respond, "Yes". Paranoia sets in as I convince myself he's found something. His silence, as he concentrates, confirms my suspicions.

Concluding his exam, he informs me, "I heard something called a bruie, or an abnormal sound in blood flow, in your abdomen. In itself, it can be harmless, and certainly many healthy people have them, but it can also result from a growth of some sort".

Continuing, he explains, "Though your medical condition may be affecting your heart, whatever is going on is not caused by the heart". In a steady, serious, soft-spoken voice, while maintaining intense, unwavering eye contact, (except for blinking), he asserts, "With the total body involvement you're presenting, you need more combined expertise than available in your local medical community. I recommend a university teaching hospital, with the benefit of a collective staff trained in diagnosing rare cases".

I respect his non-defensive honesty in admitting this case challenges the physicians I'm seeing beyond their ability. Unlike others, he does not look the other way rather than acknowledge diagnostic mistakes for what they are—but aggressively pursues treatment from a more appropriate source. Further, he assesses his own capabilities with equal objectivity, evidenced by his assertion, "Unfortunately, your symptoms don't fall within my area of expertise".

Unlike physicians who, rather than face their lack of ability to diagnose this case, told me there was nothing physically wrong, he clearly recognizes there is—but he doesn't know what. Looking into eyes that reflect security admitting he can't diagnose me, while aware of a slightly apologetic smile, I verbally lament, "Patients would respect their doctors so much more if they all exhibited your honesty." Silently, I recall how it feels to have the existence of an organic illness erroneously denied. Doctors complain that patients expect them to play God. Yet, don't they set themselves up for this role by refusing to personally accept, in their own constitutions, the basic human right of not having all the answers?

Dr. Cohen offers to discuss my case with physicians on staff at a university hospital he is associated with. Collectively, they will determine the most appropriate specialist for referral. I walk out the door feeling a little lighter, as a sense of hope pulsates through my veins for the first time in months. In an invaluable hour, this doctor managed to restore my faith in the medical profession.

Physically, this month exceeds my worst, yet. Doubled over from waves of intolerable abdominal pain so intense I can't talk through them, the excruciating cramps render the entire trunk area untouchable. With hands forced to stay at my sides at all times, it is only on rare occasions that I forget—immediately brought back to reality by an abrupt and painful reminder. If my body is the battlefield, the abdomen is clearly the front line. With each stomach cramp taking my breath away, the rhythmic surges of pain generate shivers from head-to-toe. Incessant, loud, out-of-character stomach gurgling coincides with recently increased pulsations in the area. Beyond unendurable, Dr. Michaels responds with an order for an abdominal ultrasound and a barium swallow x-ray.

Lying on the hard, metal table in a room kept uncomfortably cold, I shiver in the short-sleeved, prison-gray cotton gown I was given in exchange for my clothes. Not only do I look like an inmate, but in some respects I'm treated like one. My own thoughts, preferences and ideas are disregarded, replaced with orders I'm expected to follow unquestioningly. Basic functions are robbed of my control. I'm instructed when to breathe and when not to breathe, when to move and when to remain motionless. A technician decides my personal capacity for holding my breath, based on the frequency with which she directs me to exhale. Unfortunately, the trainee working with her doesn't always remember that "minor" detail, until my puffed out, chipmunk cheeks, (which are about to burst), loudly release air, deflating prematurely. A sheepish apology follows the forgotten instruction.

As I gulp the chalky barium mixture, (the kind of stuff you're almost afraid to taste, in spite of its intentional resemblance to a thick, tempting milkshake—but your instincts know better), reality hits. I'm nothing more than a guinea pig. After close to a year of living Hell, no one knows what is wrong with me or, more importantly, how to treat it. I endure endless process-of-elimination tests, scans and x-rays. Not only is my body abused by the disease, but by the methods used to seek diagnosis.

A physician enters the room and introduces himself. Feeling awkward attired as I am, it's fortunate, at the time, I'm unaware my lips and chin are splattered with the dried, light pink remains of the chalky mixture I've ingested. Tactfully oblivious, the doctor explains, "For the test to be most effective, we must work quickly, taking several pictures in succession. Consequently, I will be giving numerous instructions in a short period of time". Even with this warning, as I lie on the ungiving x-ray table trying to position my knee at the uncomfortable angle he requests, while struggling to drink more barium, through a flexible straw from this awkward horizontal position, the maneuvers are more difficult than I expect. Regardless, I do my best to cooperate into every contorted position required. My eyes mist as I'm again reminded of the realization that I'm nothing more than a desperate robot, automatically responding on command, with no guarantee of an answer in sight.

Dr. Cohen calls the next day, recommending a Dr. Van Deck, a rheumatologist at the university hospital he is affiliated with. Calling his office, I'm given his earliest appointment—two months away—and told to forward my medical records, which I do immediately. Optimistically, I count the days.

Checking my rural mailbox a few weeks later, I'm not surprised, among Storey's many college brochures, to receive an envelope with Dr. Van Deck's return address. I assume it is directions to his office and an appointment confirmation.

Allowing the rest of the mail to slide off my lap onto the car floor, I jaggedly tear that envelope open first, dumfounded by what I read. Dripping with sarcasm, the first line written by this doctor I've never met states, "Considering the number of highly qualified specialists you've seen, (whom he lists by name), I'm sure there's nothing I can add". The clear but unspoken implication being: because there's nothing organically wrong. "Appointment cancelled." I can't believe it—even with a doctor's referral, he refuses to see me! Hot tears of frustration sting my eyes, cooling quickly journeying their way down my cheeks, as salty droplets dry my lips. My discouragement is so profound, especially after my hopes were raised, I'm in a speechless trance. Eddie gives up trying to engage me in conversation. He knows better.

Of the many thoughts competing to outdo each other for my mind's undivided attention, the one that wins, hands down, is what am I going to do if all my doctors decide to drop me? My gut feeling tells me that Dr. Michaels, for one, would never do so. But even physicians with his patience and dedication have their limits and, undoubtedly, this case is beginning to tax them. As I pick up on understandable frustration from both him and his office staff, I ask myself if they can even begin to appreciate how frustrated I am. Feeling like the patient no doctor wants, I schedule a surgeon's appointment based on a positive gall stone report resulting from my recent x-ray.

chapter twelve

Now Do You Believe Me?

Dr. Ryan is a personal friend, selected intentionally. It's a refreshing change to go to someone I know and trust instead of being sent to specialists I've never met. And no matter how busy his schedule may be, he always makes time to fit me in.

Based on the positive ultrasound results, and pain in the area on exam, collectively we agree to gall bladder removal. The potential for eliminating this excruciating cramping is all the incentive I need. It seems almost too good to be true.

To my consternation, that's exactly what it is. Though the surgery went well, the attacks continue as forcefully as ever. Unsuccessfully trying to contend with them, in addition to my recent incision pain, tears trickle down my cheeks as I ask myself, once again, if instead of looking for a problem organ by organ, we should be addressing an entire systemic disease process that randomly attacks any, and every, organ. And if so, how am I going to get someone to really hear me?

With surgery unable to eliminate the doubling over cramping and body-wrenching chills, I spend the weekend buried under afghans, my condition worsening by the day. At Dr. Michaels' suggestion, a consult is scheduled with a rheumatologist I saw years ago, when the connective-tissue disease first surfaced. During the interim awaiting this appointment, I'm also sent to another neurologist—Dr. Ehlers. Obviously Dr. Michaels is in favor of multiple opinions, willing to seek advice anywhere if it means my getting well.

Before I'm given an opportunity to explain to Dr. Ehlers that even with surgery, the intolerable abdominal attacks continue, the doctor holds up his hand like a stop sign, telling me," I'm going to stop you short". Flipping angrily through my chart, he disgustedly throws his arms up in the air in exasperation, raising his voice as he interrupts me, interjecting, "According to your records, you've had every test known to mankind, yet no one has a clue as to what's wrong with you. You have an undiagnosable illness". From his raised negative voice the implication I hear is that there is nothing to be found. Whether it is the hopelessness he conveys, his lack of compassion, or both, I burst into tears.

Sputtering, I struggle to recover enough to coherently get out, "I can't stand this intolerable pain any longer", imploring him, "Please hospitalize me, even if only for twenty-four hours observation". Inwardly I'm convinced that if the loud, gurgling that accompanies the doubling over pain was monitored, along with the unmistakable agony registered on my ashen face, no medical professional could ethically ignore the gravity of my situation. Adamantly refusing, our first and last visit concludes.

Wiping the tears from my face, I unsuccessfully try to cover-up the fact that I've been crying before re-entering the waiting room. My swollen, road-map streaked, red eyes leave nothing to the imagination of the blank faces of waiting patients, who make no effort to hide their stares. Ignoring them, I'm pre-occupied with far more important concerns, as I leave the office feeling crushed.

Oh no, not another one of these awful attacks! I've had at least ten already today. They all start out the same way, with nauseating abdominal cramping, body-wrenching chills, and severe headache. I feel so sick I can hardly speak, let alone move. Even the slightest weight on my stomach, including that of a blanket is intolerable.

The chills come in surges, and there's nothing that stops them. Unlike those associated with a high fever, these have a buzzing sensation, almost electric-like, as they repeatedly cycle through my system. My skin is goose-bumped and my head screams with deep intense pain. It hurts so badly, I can hardly move it. Though I never know how long the headache will last, I pray it ends soon. I am rendered virtually unable to function, even minimally, until the insidious attack passes. And, unnervingly, there is no guarantee that it will. With a sigh of relief and a silent prayer, a reaction most aircraft passengers can relate to after landing safely, the attack retreats as suddenly as it came, with no way of predicting when the next one will occur.

It's been eleven years since I've seen this doctor, electing instead, Dr. Michaels, the equally competent and personable rheumatologist who has monitored my case locally. As much as I welcome the combined expertise of as many opinions as I can get, particularly from doctors I respect as much as this one, I'm immediately re-introduced to a long-since-forgotten negative aspect of this institution: it's residency training program. Before a specialist even lays eyes on a patient, the patient is involuntarily interviewed and examined by a physician-in-training.

Invariably, a want-to-be rheumatologist enters your room, introducing himself as doctor so-and-so. His assignment is to conduct a history and physical exam, the results of which he reports to the specialist with whom your appointment is scheduled. The doctor originally requested then comes in, asks additional questions and repeats the exam. In affect, the patient is subjected to multiple exams merely to facilitate the resident's training. Certainly, an ill person does not need this "benefit". Postpartum women do not need, (or want!), two pelvic exams. Patients with sore muscles and tissues shouldn't have to undergo palpitation of the same areas—twice. And no one needs excessive rectal exams!

Regretfully, the cooperating physician is often not present to oversee the doctor-in-training. As a result, it is only the patient who witnesses, at times, atrocious and inexcusable bedside manner. I've been subjected to harsh, painful exams at the hands of inexperienced and unsupervised residents. Additionally, I've been exposed to tactless interviews and undeserved disrespect. Some fire questions in rapid succession, only to rudely interrupt as the patient begins to answer them. Individuals with clear-cut diagnoses of serious ailments, with the clinical test results to corroborate them, are asked personal and insinuating questions about their marriages, whether or not they have friends, and if they are currently in therapy—by complete strangers taking advantage of a situation to sharpen their interviewing skills.

Their rushed, pre-occupied demeanor is similar to that of a student cramming for a final, lacking in sleep and unable to disguise the resulting irritability. As I think about it, there isn't much difference. Though informal, the success of their none-the-less critical exam depends on the accuracy of the findings they report to their cooperating physician.

So pressured to excel, the most desperate will go to any extreme, including cheating. After interrogating me privately as to other physicians' theories regarding my condition, I once listened in disbelief as a resident regurgitated, verbatim, the identical diagnosis to his supervisor, intentionally misleading him to believe he arrived at it independently through his exam.

Fortunately, astute cooperating physicians are aware of such tactics. I recall one, in particular, who popped his head into the exam room before sending the resident in, requesting, "Don't interpret your x-rays for the student. Lets see if he can figure them out on his own".

Recently, a resident went to summarize her findings to her cooperating physician and both returned to my room, proceeding to enter it. With one foot in the door, they began discussing my case again and retreated back into the adjacent hallway, closing the door. They then cracked it open, conversed further, shut it again, opened it about an inch and proceeded with a lengthy whispered conversation. Closing the door once more, to the muffled voices emanating from behind it, my body shivered in the skimpy, short-sleeved johnnie as I sat on the cold, hard, paper-lined table—knowing my physician and a virtual stranger-assigned resident were discussing me—and that they didn't want me to hear. How demeaning! Excuse me, but whose body is this?

My dissatisfaction with residents continues. Prior to surgery a few years ago, one was sent in to take my pre-op vital signs. When he realized the blood pressure cuff in the exam room was broken, he said, "I'll grab another before you leave". Laughingly, he added, "If I forget, I'll make up a blood pressure reading that sounds good". Well, he forgot.

When his cooperating physician reviewed my completed physical form, he questioned the blank blood pressure entry. The resident sheepishly lied, "Sorry I forgot to fill it in", quickly jotting down some numbers. God knows whose reading he recorded because it certainly wasn't mine! Fortunately for me, I was aware that my readings have always been within normal ranges, but he didn't know this. His priority was saving his own neck in the eyes of his superior, to the point that he falsified medical records. More importantly, such blatant and calculated misrepresentation could have cost a patient's life. And to think, all in the name of undue pressure placed on residents to prove their infallibility. Is it any wonder so many of them grow up to be doctors convinced they can't be wrong?

Regardless of my understandably negative impression of residents, I know that cooperating is my ticket to the specialist with whom I'm scheduled to see. Today's resident is uncomfortably serious, to the point that his face never even considers a half-smile. His lack of warmth and personable skills make for a tense interview. Then again, I'll take ability over personality any day. Nevertheless, I make a mental note to emphasize both when I someday fulfill one of my goals: teaching a course in effective doctor/patient relationships.

Scrutinizing my medical records, the impact of what he verbalizes next leaves me momentarily speechless. With a wide-eyed, open-mouthed expression of someone who's just made an unexpected and impressive discovery, followed by a look of bewilderment in my direction, he remarks, "Of course you're having these symptoms—you've had a stroke!".

Stunned immobile by his unexpected revelation, I sit statue-still, my face intentionally expressionless, silently arguing with myself that I couldn't possibly have heard right. For a moment, I thought this physician-in-training, whom I first laid eyes on not more than thirty minutes ago, just confirmed what I've known all along but couldn't prove—that I've had a stroke. But that's impossible! How could someone so inexperienced verify what renowned neurological experts missed, especially without examining me? Why, after a year of pain too severe for words, generated by extreme, yet diagnostic-defying symptoms, often dismissed by the medical profession, or worse, labeled psychosomatic, is he able to determine the cause just by talking to me?

As he traces an imaginary line with his finger under the word "ischemia" on my latest C.A.T. scan report, a repeat study I requested and Dr. Michaels ordered a couple of months ago because of continued neurological symptoms, I realize the source of his discovery. Ironically, it is the only result not yet included in my own personal file of medical records. As he continues, I barely hear a word he's saying. My mind is stuck on the word "stroke". How could such a neurological disaster have gone undetected until now? It's not like it just occurred. It happened the night I saw those lights. Without warning, my world transformed so dramatically, I felt like I entered another galaxy. Yet I consulted so many specialists since that regrettable incident. Why didn't anyone pick up on it? And, when I proposed the possibility, why did they dismiss it so vehemently? Did I suffer unendurable symptoms, needlessly, for a year because of medical community close-mindedness? If so, and at this point, what else am I to believe, it's a pathetic commentary on medical credibility in the 1990's.

No wonder the resident gave me such a perplexed look! He's probably wondering why I didn't just come out and tell him I've had a stroke, instead of listing all the symptoms of one, as if diagnosis is a mystery. Considering the scan was done two months ago, he makes the logical assumption that, by now, I've been informed of the abnormality—but, in fact, I haven't. Little does he know, as he begins the physical exam, that he's the first doctor to confirm the diagnosis I've suspected all along, or how grateful I am to him for doing so.

Appreciative as I am, I'm unwilling to admit surprise over his revelation. As difficult as it is for me to explain why, I guess it comes down to principle. Unofficially, I've known all along I've had a stroke. It's the only thing that could account for such bizarre and overnight changes. I've lived the repercussions of that trauma every agonizing minute, of every day, since the incident. There have been countless sleepless nights, lying on a saturated pillow sobbing in silent darkness, except for the rhythmic breathing of my husband, as he sleeps peacefully beside me. No matter how many people loved me and sincerely empathized with this nightmare, it was mine and mine, alone. There are no words strong enough to describe the private kind of Hell I lived. Sheer desperation no legitimately ill patient deserves to know forced me to pursue an answer to this madness on my own. I'm not about to give someone else credit for this diagnosis.

Suddenly, I'm consumed with anger so intense, every blood vessel encased in this adrenaline-ignited body threatens to burst. Extreme heat surges through each cell, with fever-like penetration. While my escalating rage isn't directed at the resident, himself, it does target others in the profession he represents. Mentally reliving unforgettable episodes from the year long medical battle I was forced to wage, I'm appalled by the inexcusably poor treatment I encountered.

How dare these so-called, dedicated professionals tell a stroke victim nothing neurological happened? And, as if denying such a serious medical reality isn't enough, to recommend that she see a psychiatrist for residual symptoms, which these egocentric, self-proclaimed infallible physicians refused to recognize as such, is deplorable. Stroke patients require immediate medical attention—not rejection from physicians.

I should have been hospitalized and placed on a stroke watch and recovery program. Much of the overwhelming fear of the unknown could have been prevented if someone explained to me why, virtually overnight, I felt like a complete stranger had taken up residence in the shell of my former self. If only someone could have confirmed the neurological accident responsible for my bizarre symptoms, I would've accepted it.

Instead, out of desperation, I self-diagnosed, predicting worse case scenarios. With the persistence of someone fighting for her life, which I truly believe I am, I launched a campaign of letter writing, phone calling and doctor-hopping, driven to exhaust every potential for an answer to this nightmare. Letters go unanswered, phone calls unreturned and appointments unscheduled as one specialist after another dismisses my case. Unfortunately, though the few who stick by me provide emotional support, they are unable to alleviate my physical symptoms.

The consequences of too many physicians failing me, once too often, is the irreparable loss of credibility in a profession I once trusted. While my body screams from the physical abuse, resulting from untreated symptoms allowed to run rampant, my head screams from emotional abuse. At a point in time when I require medical expertise more than ever, I'm hesitant to trust again. The memory of this demeaning diagnostic fiasco is still too fresh in my mind—and the emotional scars too deep.

My mind is in overdrive, recalling one rationalization after another, used to label my symptoms anything but, stroke-related. From hyperventilation, to anxiety, to migraines, to steroid-psychosis, to depression, the list goes on. My face flushes warmth with a renewed surge of anger as I recall one physician's description of me as "a person who looks far healthier than I claim to feel". With rising heat that continues to infiltrate my body, I relive the unforgettable specialist's appointment during which I was told the specific dollar amount "wasted" on my testing only to reveal that I'm "perfectly fine". And how dare a neurologist dismiss life-threatening symptoms as nothing more than a "phobia" resulting from having seen lights?

I can still feel the emotional sting of the hand-slapping admonishment by the doctor who advised me to "stop causing your husband unnecessary worry, maintaining you're ill when you're not". Informing me "not to purchase a cemetery plot", this same neurologist became visibly irritated and sarcastic with me at the mere inquiry as to whether I could have had a stroke. Equally damaging, one of his peers at another university insisted I didn't need a neurologist; instead, I needed a "good psychiatrist". There are no words to adequately describe how it felt to be so desperately ill—and not heard. Virtually every stroke symptom I reported was undermined, rationalizing each to a much less serious origin.

During the indescribably horrific diagnostic process, my personal efforts toward resolution were regarded unfavorably. I was criticized for logging a handwritten list of symptoms and cited negatively for acquired medical terminology and understanding. The unmistakable implication was that it enabled me to continue this "pretense" of being ill. With few exceptions, I felt ignored, demeaned and left to fend for myself by condescending physicians who, often subjectively, denied the gravity of my condition.

Neurologists aware of effective medications to treat nausea and dizziness offered none. Convinced no physical illness existed, they angrily turned me away, vehemently insisting, "You're seeing the wrong kind of doctor!". When I reached the point that I awakened suppressing the urge to vomit every time I turned in my sleep, I requested an antivert derivative, with which Dr. Michaels, not one of the neurologists, complied. In retrospect, I should have been on it since the stroke, given the immediate relief it provided.

My unspoken, inner tirade is interrupted when the resident, completing his exam, informs me, "I'll be back in a few minutes with Dr. Ames". Left alone in the exam room, I review the results of the C.A.T. scan, which are on the desk. In speechless horror, I read a notation to the affect that the stroke may have been present at the time of my original scan, almost a year ago, but, due to "technical problems", may not have been read as such.

To think, so much pain and doctor-hopping could have been avoided if I was diagnosed accurately back then! Not to mention humiliation. Just as the reality of what this oversight really meant in my life begins to sink in, Dr. Ames and the resident enter the room. It takes a concerted effort to greet her congenially and discuss how long it's been since we last saw each other. My mind rages a silent battle over the ineptitude of so many representatives of her profession.

Within minutes, her genuine warmth and sincere concern, qualities I respected in her when we first met years ago, win over my preoccupation. Somehow, this dedicated woman exudes caring just by entering a room. Whether it's the concern registered in her warm, compassionate eyes, the tenderness of her voice, her effective listening skills or a combination of all three, she easily earns the respect of her patients, myself included.

Confirming that my symptoms are stroke-related, she advises me to remain in the care of a neurologist. Additionally, she recommends that, if I'm not already doing so, I should take an aspirin a day, without fail, as a stroke preventative. I leave silently grateful that I independently instituted this therapy, months ago, when I first suspected a stroke.

chapter thirteen
Surprise Visitor

Not again! No! I refuse to accept it. After finally obtaining a clinical diagnosis that logically explains the horrific nightmare I've been living, physicians can't be questioning the validity of this scan, too. Yet, incredibly, they are.

A follow-up study, read by a different radiologist, failed to interpret a stroke. I love it! My life is on the line and effective treatment is dependent upon the subjectivity of the physicians reviewing the films. The fact that I've been complaining of every stroke symptom known to man, including numbness, slurred speech, blurry vision, swallowing difficulty, weakness, dizziness and headaches, is disregarded. What are they going to do, wait until I have a massive stroke before they believe me? And if so, how will they justify that, to Eddie and the girls, knowing I've been warning them all along?

With stroke confirmation now debatable between two radiologists, the tests, scans and even surgeries continue. I'm so desperately ill at this point, I'll agree to anything that offers even the slightest hope of diagnosis and treatment—including the role of a guinea pig.

As Stacey prepares for mid-term exams, I intentionally try to camouflage my health. We're so connected, that to do otherwise could preoccupy her to the point of adverse performance on her tests.

It takes concerted effort to appear up-beat whenever she calls. Trying to sound cheerful, while experiencing an excruciating headache, can be impossible. And, on a few occasions, I'm less convincing than I'd like. When I am, I address her perceptive questions, delivered in an unmistakable panicked voice, that gets higher as her anxiety builds, with the excuse that I'm tired. Her relieved sigh, audible long-distance as I provide this rationale, assures me she suspects nothing, particularly when she animatedly proceeds to share, with typical Stacey exuberance, aspects of her relatively carefree life.

Doing my best to concentrate on speaking smoothly, I fight the natural inclination of my chill-wracked body to formulate stuttering syllables. Through chattering teeth, I continue my personal guilt-provoking act.

The well-intentioned facade is becoming increasingly difficult to maintain, however. Stacey knows me too well. She not only picks up suspicious clues in my voice, but she interrogates her less-deceptive sister, and her friends, regarding my health status. This, coupled with the noticeable decrease in daily letters she customarily receives from me, provides more information about my condition than I care to share—and she's worried.

The excuse that my eyes are hurting is no longer convincing. She knows how much I enjoy writing to her and that I'd do so regardless if my eyes ached. The truth of the matter is there are days on which I have difficulty seeing the lines on the paper. The letters fade in and out. Sometimes I only see every other one, with shadows making them unclear. My customarily typewriter-neat, elementary school teacher printing is now barely discernible.

Within the next few weeks, Stacey's regular phone calls home increase to one a day. She's onto me. When she calls me and confronts me point-blank, I can't lie to her. "Mom, I want the truth. I just got a call at school from Michelle, (her best friend). She said I must really be scared. According to her, the whole town is worried about you. I knew you weren't feeling well when you saw those lights but have things gotten worse?" With a resigned sigh, I admit, "Yes, Stacey, I'm ill—very ill". "Mom, what's wrong with you?", her voice quivers. "No one seems to know for sure" I reply. "All I know is I've never felt so sick in my entire life". "Can't they do anything?", she pleads. "We're trying, Stacey", I say in a voice that lacks conviction. "Mom, you're scaring me. I'm closer to you than anyone in the whole world. No one understands me like you do", her voice cracks. "I know, honey, and believe me, I'm fighting with every ounce of strength I have." In a tender moment we share tears, long-distance, while a much-needed hug is put on hold.

I have mixed feelings about Stacey knowing. I regret that she's pre-occupied worrying about me. Yet, I welcome the support from someone I've missed confiding in. By the time our warm, compassionate and long-overdue conversation ends, I'm convinced leveling with her was the right thing to do. Besides, the last time she saw me I put on a very convincing act. I can no longer pull that off. This conversation was essential to prepare her for what to expect when classes adjourn for mid-semester break next month.

I'm not the mom she came home to at Christmas, not that I was myself, then. But by the day, I grow worse. I spend much of my time wrapped cocoon-like in several afghans, unsuccessfully trying to over-compensate for the unrelenting waves of chills throughout the day and night. I rarely drive, except when no one else is available. I've stopped eating out at restaurants, something I once enjoyed. I'm drawn and listless. The person I've become is a far cry from the one I was. I don't even know her, much less what to expect next from this stranger.

I even look different. I've never been so thin in my entire adult life. Ordinarily, I'd be thrilled. But this new body, transformed without conscious dieting, is just one more indication of how sick I really am. As my rib cage prominently displays its bony structure, I intentionally avoid mirrors. Will this madness ever stop? And what if it doesn't?

My physician is understandably concerned. For the first time in my life, I've been instructed to gain weight. In reading my copies of physicians' letters to other doctors, I'm referred to as "thin". Who could they be talking about? Certainly not the person who, for years, envied people who could eat anything and not gain a pound.

Lying in bed negatively assessing the new me, I'm immediately jolted out of my pessimism as Stacey pops her head through the bedroom doorway, the unexpected visit a total shock. Her cursory, but unmistakable scrutiny of my changed image, as we rush into each others' arms, leaves me silently thanking God that I prepared her ahead of time.

My eyes fill to hear her explain, "I borrowed money and took two buses home, transferring in New York City. Michelle's parents picked me up at the bus terminal in Hartford. I just had to see you." "But, honey, aren't you in the middle of exams?", the mother part of me asks, without hiding my need to hug her tighter. "Don't worry, mom. I brought my books home. Actually, I'll probably get more studying done here than in my noisy dorm."

Though momentarily shocked to see her, as I think about it, I shouldn't be. That's the type of person Stacey is—warm and caring. Throw in a bit impulsive, much like her mom, and it's no surprise she's here this weekend. Regardless of how she got home, what caused her to do it when instead, she should be studying for exams, or how she's getting back, all I care about at the moment is that she's here. And I need her.

I'm determined to make this weekend as positive as possible, starting with doing my best to allay the intense fear which I realize precipitated this unannounced visit at such a busy time in her academic schedule. Beginning to prepare some of her favorite foods, grateful that I have the ingredients on hand, I do my best to ignore the intense dizziness whenever I stand. I attempt to counteract the weakness by leaning most of my weight against the kitchen counter, much like I do at the bathroom sink when I brush my teeth. The weakest part of me is my legs. They feel so heavy, like they could be swallowed up by the floor if I don't hold onto something.

Throughout the weekend, I catch Stacey staring at me pensively. I particularly notice it as I tuck a shirt into my jeans. As soon as she realizes I observe her scrutinizing me, she quickly covers up with a complimentary comment, "Someone's lost weight". Yet, her look is one of unmistakable worry.

Explaining she needs to go to the mall for about an hour, (unwilling to sacrifice more study time than that), to purchase a birthday gift for a friend, she hesitantly asks, "Would you like to come?". The doubt in her eyes, and the sheepish expression on her face, tells me she predicts a negative answer and that inviting me was just wishful thinking on her part. I don't have the heart to say no. Besides, I'm scared. Driven by an insidious inner nagging to do as much as I can, while I can, my actions are controlled in more ways than I'd like since the onset of this madness. "I'd love to", I respond automatically.

During the ride, my view from the passenger's seat is blurry signs and scenery, intensifying my nausea with each mile we travel. As Stacey animatedly describes college life and how much she's enjoying it, I have all I can do to concentrate on what she is saying. I'm sitting within two feet of her, yet I feel so far away and removed. It's like we're not even in the same car—and that her voice is an echo in the distance.

By the time we arrive at the mall, I'm so nauseated I can hardly stand, let alone walk around shopping with her. Using the excuse that I have things to look for, as well, I suggest separating to consolidate time. Instead, I find a seat in the food court. Amid a blur of happy faces, excitedly describing their purchases to lunchtime companions in the filled-to-capacity eatery, I sit consumed by an intense headache, miserably counting the minutes until she returns.

I can't believe how fast this weekend flew by. Getting into the car as we prepare to take Stacey to her bus terminal, two hours away, I'm overcome with weakness in my right leg which buckles, threatening to collapse. Insecure, what are customarily automatic movements, become calculated. Intentionally electing not to share this unnerving development with my family, I find myself testing leg strength, discreetly, throughout the car ride. Undeniably, there is a decided difference between the two. I can't lift the right one an inch off the floor without it shaking uncontrollably. Just as I'm beginning to wonder if this bus terminal really exists, a fleet of streamlined silver, parked equidistant to each other, glistening in the bright sun, comes into view.

Tenuously getting out of the car, I'm afraid to test my weight on my weak leg. Instead, I precariously distribute it between the left leg and the door. The car retaliates loudly with a noisy creak, unaccustomed to supporting adult weight with its passenger door.

To the overpowering smell of diesel polluting the air, we learn we consulted the wrong schedule. Stacey's bus left hours ago. Resigned to wait for the next one, due in two hours, we decide to go to lunch.

According to Eddie and Stacey, the food at the nearby restaurant is excellent, living up to the billboard advertisement that originally attracted us. Given today's lack of appetite, nothing from their varied menu appealed. Relenting to my family's warning that I have to eat if I expect to maintain enough strength to fight off whatever is going on, I order a cheeseburger, managing only a few bites.

As I get up to use the ladies room, the leg weakness is so pronounced, I'm especially grateful for the mid-afternoon, non-prime dining time. The virtually desolate room allows me to unselfconsciously grab onto each empty table I pass, inching my way to the bathroom. Once there, I feel even more insecure because no one else is in the room and I sense I'm going to fall. Breaking out into a fear-induced sweat, I exit as quickly as my weak appendage allows, joining Eddie and Stacey in the car.

During the short ride to the bus stop, there is uncharacteristic silence. I'm afraid to say good-bye to Stacey. I no longer interpret this common departure word as the nonchalant "see you later" it is intended to mean. Instead, an uncertain future ominously assigns it foreboding finality. I sense Stacey shares my reluctance to say good-bye. In spite of my concerted efforts to cover-up this weekend, she's witnessed too much. There are some things one just can't hide, especially from someone so emotionally connected.

Quickly getting out of the car, she utters an artificially cheerful "good-bye"—too cheerful under the circumstances—and rushes toward the terminal. That, in itself, is atypical of Stacey. She never leaves without a hug. Unwilling to forego the affection I'm accustomed to, especially now, as pessimistic scenarios I'd prefer not to face project their ugly images on the big screen in my mind with unrelenting insensitivity, I call after her, my voice cracking from undisguised emotion, "Stacey don't leave without a hug".

Through the wavy, distorted vision of tears brimming to fall, I look into the glossy blue pools of Stacey's eyes. This particular departure is especially painful to both of us. Neither knows what to expect when we see each other again—or, if we will, for that matter. And we're both scared.

Eddie embraces our tearful daughter, "Do well on your exams, hon", comes the loving, wishful-thinking piece of parental advice, uttered more for the thought itself than the reality that she will be able to concentrate under such adverse circumstances. Waiting for her call later that night, to say she arrived safely, I'm saddened but not surprised to learn that she cried the entire return bus trip. Unsuccessfully blinking back tears of my own, I ask myself if any mother could possibly love their children as much as I do mine.

Snuggled between our warm, cozy flannel sheets, covered with a matching hand-stitched quilt, we're contentedly oblivious to the record-breaking, frigid February chill the T.V. weatherman reports. Instead, we remain right where we are, comfortably absorbed in a movie. At one point, the leading actor tells his significant other that she is his hope for happiness. Lightheartedly, Eddie takes my hand, nonchalantly repeating those words to me. Without warning, and as much of a shock to me as to Eddie, I burst into tears, blubbering inconsolably, "You shouldn't allow your happiness to depend on me".

It's what I don't say—but can't help thinking—that makes me cry even harder. Convinced I'm a poor risk, I'm terrified I'm dying. I certainly don't want his happiness to end if I do. I want so much more for him. He deserves so much more. Though I don't put my fears into words, I don't have to. Eddie knows exactly what I'm thinking as he embraces my sob-induced, convulsing body, whispering comforting words into my ear. The suspicion that I might not always be here for him and our girls is not mine alone. I can tell by the way he watches me so closely, lately, that he is preoccupied with his own, unspoken fears. He's scared. We all are. Living with an illness that ravages one's body insidiously is tenuous at best. The daily insecurity of an uncertain future, and its potential ramifications to one's family, is a kind of hell only someone who has lived it can know. Is it any wonder my emotions are so on edge, lately? I keep telling myself if I knew what to expect I'd learn to deal with it. But I don't—no one does.

chapter fourteen
She's Not a Kid Anymore

As I hang up the phone, I'm pre-occupied with the revelation that I'm in parental denial and have been right along. Like so many mothers, though my children are growing into mature adults right before my eyes, there's a part of me that chooses not to see it. Overprotection certainly factors into my subconscious resistance to acknowledge the natural maturation process, as does the unwillingness to let go of them, yet. Instead, I observe adults-in-the-making in my friends' children, as they go off to college a little unsure of their independent venture, only to return for Christmas break confident and with direction. I'm sure my friends saw this in Stacey. I didn't, or more to the point, chose not to—until now.

Caught off guard when she called to say she was bringing someone home for us to meet, my initial reaction was why is she even telling us? During the two years she has been a student at an upstate New York university, we've welcomed and encouraged her weekend guests with or without notice.

My momentary confusion, the result of naive denial, was abruptly replaced with a reality check when, in her next breath, she explained, "My friend is a guy". Swallowing the hard, dry, saliva-deficient lump that sticks in one's throat when taken by complete surprise, I feel like I'm attempting to down a moistureless wad of cotton.

Overnight, whether I'm ready to accept it or not, (because fate doesn't take that into consideration), the adorable baby girl whose birth, nineteen years ago, left me in speechless awe, grew up. Listening to her confident, excited voice, registering decibels higher than usual, on the other end of the phone, I nostalgically contrast to when, as a child, she depended on me for everything.

Part of me isn't ready to believe that this is the same kid who, only months old, clung to me desperately as I held her close to my chest, reassuring her that everything was okay during mom and tot swim classes. My memory can still resurrect the sweet aroma of her baby breath as she positioned her face close to mine, focused on my every word. Though too young to understand their meaning, the recognizable tone provided security.

And what mother can't recall that magic moment when their child released their crumpled up little fist from around her finger and gingerly, almost drunken-like, took that very first step alone? I don't know whose eyes were wider, mine or Stacey's, when we realized she had actually done it!

As the milestones in her life continue to flashback through my mind, I smile recalling her initial hesitancy to sit on Santa's lap. Little did she know, "Santa" was an uncle she adored. One of my favorite memories is totally surprising her for her sixth birthday with a trip to Disney World. Eddie videotaped her excitement as she read her card out loud, describing the gift, including the part where she jumped up and down, asking us to "Pinch me to prove I'm not dreaming". Her eyes grew so wide, on this seasonably cold February evening, to learn her summer clothes were already packed and in the car, in anticipation of our early morning flight.

Where did the years go? I feel like I blinked my eyes and she went from diapers to dates. I'm again reminded of the lyrics, "This is the Time to Remember, For it Will Not Last Forever". I wasn't ready to accept it as we dropped her off at college and a part of me isn't ready to believe it now.

But ready or not, the time has come. My reaction is important to Stacey. Without further hesitation, and as casually as I can make myself sound under the circumstances, I respond, "We'd love to meet your friend". Stacey knows me far too well to fall for my out-of-character nonchalance, however. Her knowing, suspicious laugh tells me she sees right through it. Rescuing me as I fight the urge to bombard her with the universally-nosy questions reserved just for mothers, at times such as this, she fills me in on the details. Before our conversation ends, I learn that she and Tim met several months ago at a college party. "And, yes, he's the guy who called me at home, in Connecticut, over Christmas break", she admits for the first time, even though she knew I was dying of curiosity when the original call was made. "He is from upstate New York, a senior in college, graduating this May." Commenting further that she's "sure he is someone you and dad will like a lot", of this I have no doubt. Stacey has always exercised good judgment in her choice of friends, never bringing home anyone even the slightest bit questionable, in our minds.

The feeling she doesn't verbalize, and probably the most important, is the message I read loud and clear between the lines: This guy is someone very special to her. Of the people she's dated at college, he is the first she's asked to bring home. It doesn't even take that extra sense, that all mothers instinctively possess, to recognize that this is different. Clearly, she's looking for her family's opinion and, hopefully, approval. With mixed emotions, fluctuating between feeling slightly threatened that she might have found someone more special than us to enter her world, and sincere excitement for her, I begin preparing the special meal she requested.

As I saute the onions for the French Onion Soup, I'm overwhelmed by nauseating, doubling-over stomach cramps. The pain is so bad I can barely stand. Hunching my way over to the table, I crumple into a chair and begin to pray, "Please God not now. Not at this important stage in Stacey's life. Let me be okay for this weekend. Don't let me spoil it."

The pain continues. Unfortunately, I don't have the luxury of even a few minutes time to waste. I've got too much to get done before they come home. I feel so sick—like I could just keel over and die. (Though in reality I don't know what one feels like at such a time, I can't imagine feeling worse than this.) But I will myself to keep going. I refuse to let this nightmare interfere with the things I'm determined to do. I didn't fight this hard, for this long, to give up now.

Who am I trying to kid? I look just awful. My eyes are bloodshot and my skin is pasty white. My expression is intense, no doubt the result of this unrelenting pain. My reflection is so unnerving to me that I avoid mirrors, lately. Denial is not an option, however. I don't have to look at myself to realize how gravely ill I am. All I have to do is live the pain raging inside of me. And, at the moment, I have no alterative.

Doing my best to accomplish the impossible, camouflaging the telltale signs of severe internal illness, which insidiously register across my face like a neon sign flashing SICK in capital letters, I apply some blush. Stubbornly, my eerie, ghostlike complexion rejects even artificial pigmentation. Regardless of how thickly I layer it on, I look anemic. My hope is that Stacey will be too distracted by Tim's presence to notice. The deceptively ferocious bark of Paddington, who on occasion has been known to retreat into his doghouse, frightened by a little turtle, tells me I'm about to find out.

The deep voice and tall stature that accompanies Stacey into our home serves as another reality check. I don't know what I was expecting but, one thing is certain, Tim is no boy. At twenty-three, extending his outstretched hand securely to Eddie, who eagerly greets him, he is the first man she's brought home. Boys are the guys she went to her proms with. The difference is standing in my kitchen watching me, as I try to ignore the butterflies in my stomach, while attempting to pull off the calm, Harriet Nelson look at the stove. As this clean-cut looking guy, the type that every mother dreams her daughter will bring home, greets me, relief surges through my body. By the end of the weekend, having had the opportunity to get to know Tim a little better, and observe firsthand how effectively he and Stacey interact, I'm even more grateful that they met.

chapter fifteen

Do My Doctors Realize What They Expect of Me?

On this Sunday morning in late April, as I lie in bed listening to the birds chirp, the warmth of the sun's rays streaking through the curtains reminds me that it's finally beyond flannel sheet time. I was beginning to think this day would never come. Following a horrendous winter, with record-breaking snows, so far the first month of spring has been anything but promising. From the looks of today, that's about to change.

Making a mental note to switch to more seasonally appropriate bed linens, less optimistic thoughts begin cluttering my mind, at such a pace that I decide I'd better write them down before I lose them. It's not as though it hasn't happened before. It seems I do my most descriptive, creative thinking while lying in bed, only to be stored in irretrievable memory banks of my mind by the time I attempt to document them hours later.

I can't afford to let that happen this time. The ominous undertone of today's thoughts trouble me. As intolerable symptoms increase by the day, with no diagnosis in sight, I allow my mind to entertain the unnerving fear that unless something is done soon, I stand to lose my sanity. Ironically, I don't think my physicians have a clue as to how close I am.

They've repeatedly listened to me describe the physical ramifications but have they really heard me? Is there any way they can appreciate the panic initiated by the suffocating sensation that jars me out of my sleep, desperately gasping for life-sustaining air? Can they even begin to understand what it is like to experience sustained visual deterioration, with letters fading out or impossible to read, with no explanation? Or urinary incontinence, indescribably severe headaches and numbness throughout my body?

Are there any words to more clearly convey the drunken-like stupor that now constitutes my being? Though I've tried to describe the tipsy, room-swimming way in which I view the world, unless one looks through my eyes, it is impossible to comprehend.

My physicians are expecting too much of me. My symptoms are terrifying—far too frightening to face alone. Their systemic nature, with every organ and system throughout my body involved, only adds to the gravity of my condition.

My body is failing me fast and I'm desperate for someone to acknowledge that fact and treat these unnerving, and potentially life-threatening symptoms, aggressively. I'm needy for someone out there to hear me. The irony is although I'm at a physical stage where I can't afford to expend precious energy pursuing this seemingly hopeless effort, I can't afford not to.

Beyond that, I have a right to know what is going on. It's my body—and my life. If I have something treatable, then let's get started, I can only hope this inexcusable delay doesn't mean it's too late. If, on the other hand, what I have is not treatable, I have a right to know that, too. Should I be in a terminal situation, I deserve the option of Hospice. It's not my choice to go this alone. In this day in age one shouldn't have to. Yet, it seems that every desperate attempt I make to get help is stifled. At this rate, I pray I'm alive to see this book in print.

Anger ignites every cell in my body, like a fever raging from head-to-toe, whenever my doctors advise me to "keep going". The more I hear these empty words, the more control it takes to suppress the urge to scream. A meaningless statement, void of any hope and compassion, offering no treatment plan to cling to, mouthed more for the benefit of making the physician, himself, feel better. But have they stopped to consider what they're asking me to do? If experiencing the same symptoms, could they "keep going"?

The unlikelihood of that probability stimulates my mind to conjure up a scenario of a physician practicing under such adverse circumstances. The exhausted doctor is late for his first appointment because he can no longer drive and his ride wasn't on time. With dark-circled, expressionless eyes, a drawn face and a dramatic weight loss, he looks far more ill than his patient. His interview skills are inadequate because his mind is less sharp from lack of sleep. Complicating it more, he hears his patient speaking but he feels "unconnected", as though very far away and unable to concentrate. Fortunately, the patient is cooperative and repeats himself as often as the doctor makes the request.

On the way to the exam room, the physician stumbles into the wall. Unsure of whether blurry vision or dizziness caused it, the result is the same. When he finally steadies his tremoring hand enough to shine a light in his patient's eyes, he can't focus on them because his own eyes gray out. Discreetly, he uses the sleeve of his lab coat to wipe drool from the side of his mouth. His suddenly sunburned-looking face is the only telltale sign of the clammy urinary incontinence that just occurred. Fortunately, he had the foresight to take precautions when he dressed that morning so that his secret remains intact. Hopefully, the patient will assume it is the heat of the radiator in the exam room that made him color.

It's a good thing the bandaids were recently replenished. He never expected that involuntary jerk of his right hand, while holding a glass slide. If only his assistant had been standing on his left side, instead. Oh well, it could have been worse. Her hand only required one of those small, round bandages. You know, the kind that identify and decorate the faces of men who got up late and rushed through shaving.

Since the assistant administers the patient's E.K.G., it is strategically planned for when the physician needs to run to the bathroom, doubled over with cramps. That way, his quick exit is less conspicuous. When he is delayed for several minutes beyond the completion of the heart tracing, his tactful, albeit somewhat dishonest assistant, explains he must be on the phone. It had to be some conversation judging from the anemic complexion that accompanies him back to the exam room! Though he gives the patient a clean bill of health, she's not sure if she heard right because his speech is so slurred. For a moment, she wonders if he might be an alcoholic, or on drugs, especially considering the stressful profession he is in. She immediately dismisses that theory, not wanting to entertain such thoughts about her doctor.

Instead, she tells him he doesn't seem himself and suggests he make an appointment for an evaluation. Though on the surface, it appears that he takes her advice when he schedules the appointment, it is really something he'd been planning to do for quite some time.

What a relief to hear that his tests are all normal and that he has a clean bill of health! Just to be told by someone he holds in such high esteem, that there is nothing blatantly wrong, is reassuring in itself. As the physician leaves his doctor's office, he smiles on his way out when his doctor advises him to "keep going". Unfortunately, that's exactly what he did.

That's the last anyone heard from him. Rumor has it he lost his mind and still hasn't found it.

This ludicrously hypothetical illustration demonstrates more truth than immediately meets the eye. Doctors who don't recognize their patients' pain, and address it constructively, jeopardize far more than their comfort. Reflecting on the number of incompetent physicians who refused to interact, medically, on my behalf, I'm consumed with anger so intense that bulging veins ripple my skin, visibly popping to the surface. If it were in my power, I'd revoke the medical license of every doctor who has turned me away. Anyone capable of refusing treatment to the seriously ill doesn't deserve to practice medicine.

A couple of hours ago, I learned of another patient who, like me, registered ischemia on a C.A.T. scan. Her neurological symptoms continued, undiscouraged, until she dropped dead of a massive stroke—the same thing my paternal grandmother died from. Is that what has to happen to me before I earn the respect of the medical community? Is preventative medicine, a catch phrase of physicians in the nineties, merely lip service? Sadly, I've become the victim of egocentric doctoring. Rather than admit to gross initial misdiagnosis of this case, my continued and desperate pleas for help fall on deaf ears, with each day I remain untreated threatening my life further. And the irony is, this patient who has everything to live for, is powerless to stop it from happening. Like an innocent victim of a fatal car crash, I, too, can be right—dead right!

Dear Family:

When God gave me a husband and daughters, he gave me the best—and if having the "best" meant living with this illness, I'd do it all over again to have each of you. I say this because of the quality of our relationships. I wouldn't trade my family for the world—and I know you feel the same about me. You taught me a definition of love that reached a depth I never knew until each of you came into my life. I thank God for all of you because, to me, you're what love is all about.

Know that I'm desperately fighting this illness—and have been, right along. Regardless of the outcome, the three of you are my best incentives toward beating this thing. And I'm not a quitter!

Love,
Mom

An eye exam the following week reveals decreased blood flow to the optic nerve. No wonder I'm experiencing neurological problems—my brain isn't getting enough oxygen! In retrospect, had this abnormality shown up sooner, back when I initially sought medical attention for blurry vision and other stroke-suspicious developments, I probably wouldn't have been dismissed by some of the best neurologists in the country. But it's unproductive to dwell on that now. Besides, I have far more important things to concentrate on.

As the symptoms associated with this alarming, and until now, undiagnosed oxygen deprivation increase and intensify, unrestrained, by the day, it doesn't require a medical degree to predict another stroke waiting to happen. What other signs do my physicians need before initiating aggressive, pro-active treatment? Considering the unnerving potential for irreversible brain damage if a major neurological accident should occur, I owe it to myself to do whatever I can to try to prevent one. Though there may be nothing I, as a lay person, can do to alter an unavoidable eventuality, Eddie, Stacey and Storey are reason enough to at least try.

Out of desperation, and at loss as to where else to begin, I head for our local library to research addresses of major medical institutions throughout The United States. As I strain to focus my blurry vision on the small print entries in the directory I consult, it occurs to me that this shouldn't be my job. I'm far too ill to expend precious energy pursuing a diagnosis of my own. Yet too many medical specialists have turned deaf and/or close-minded ears to my cries for help, leaving me no recourse.

Though they've run tests, I see these efforts as attempts to pacify me, temporarily getting me off their backs, yet stopping before diagnosis, as each reaches their frustration point. For the long, painful weeks and months between procedures, I'm on my own unsuccessfully dealing with excruciating symptoms that won't quit. Immediate, aggressive treatment to attack the life-threatening, systemic war raging out-of-control within my body, is essential. Selecting several well-known institutions, I direct the following plea for help to the heads of their Neurology and Rheumatology Departments:

To Whom It May Concern:

The purpose of this letter is to acquaint the physicians at your facility with a medical condition that, to date, remains undiagnosed. It is my hope, and that of my primary care physician, that after reading this synopsis letter, your institution will consider evaluation of this case.

Following ten years of mixed connective-tissue disease involvement, which manifested itself in muscle and joint pain, oral and nasal ulcers, Raynoud's phenomenon, facial rashes and abnormal thyroid levels, in March of 1994, this illness took on a more serious slant.

Within minutes of an episode in which I saw clear, continuous, multi-faceted lights that cascaded toward me, I began experiencing extreme changes throughout my entire body. These included stabbing pins-and-needles, swallowing difficulty, complete loss of appetite, "novocaine-numb" limbs, tingling, forceful involuntary muscle jerking, (which jolt my husband and I out of a sound sleep), severe, frequent headaches, nausea, dizziness, blurred vision, transient urinary incontinence, a disassociated feeling, (distant and removed, a faraway sensation), and a significant increase in the momentary "rippling" sensation, (almost like liquid pulsating, that I've had since the onset of the connective-tissue disease). In addition, at times I drool out of one side of my mouth or tear from one eye. All of these symptoms commenced immediately following the lights' incident and have continued ever since.

To date, I've had an abnormal S.P.E.C.T. scan, a C.A.T. scan which indicated ischemia, a sleep study that recorded one hundred and fifty muscle jerk awakatures within four hours, and an aberrant split-screen E.E.G. I have been unable to detect cold instruments from my thighs to my feet, across my forehead and from my hands to my elbows. Nystagmus was observed on exam.

To conclude, due to the severity of these symptoms, your input would be appreciated by both myself and my physician. We look forward to your earliest response and the potential for a consult appointment in the near future.

Thank you in advance for your consideration.

Sincerely,

Eileen Radziunas

chapter sixteen
Cape Cod

As weeks turn to months, the symptoms multiply while the pain intensifies. It becomes increasingly difficult to maintain my busy schedule but, for all our sakes,—I must.

Pulling into the parking lot on this stiflingly oppressive July day, I intentionally park under the shadiest tree I can find. Waiting for Storey's National Honor Society meeting to adjourn, even with the windows all the way down, there isn't a breeze to be had in the stagnant, almost too-thick-to-breathe, humid air. Sweat-induced ringlets transform my normally wavy hair into an Afro as my clothes stick uncomfortably to me.

The parking lot is relatively desolate, compared to when school is in session. Those that do come and go reflect the summer setting: office employees dressed in casual shorts outfits, a student returning a softball uniform now that the season is over, two toddlers and their mom visiting the principal, (a relative with whom they have a takeout food picnic), and a lone student biking leisurely through the lot. The absence of any National Honor Society students exiting the building confirms what Storey warned me of when suggesting a time to pick her up—the meeting might go a lot longer than her estimate.

To the sounds of birds chirping a language no interpreter could begin to understand, fuzzy, green, viney droppings silently drift from an overhead tree, tickling my exposed arm. Giving in to overwhelming fatigue, the peaceful setting induces me to sleep. A sudden forceful, involuntary jerk of my left foot jolts me awake. Frightened by the violent intrusion, I note the dashboard clock is only five minutes later than when I last looked.

Over the past month, these catnaps have become the norm, the result of depleted energy from the incredulous amount of inexcusable legwork I, personally, have had to expend toward seeking medical intervention. Since seeing those lights, I've asked nothing more of my physicians than the serious treatment my condition requires—and I deserve. With few exceptions, my needs have been ignored. As a result, I'm experiencing Medical Hell at the hands of professionals I once trusted. There are no words strong enough to convey how it feels to be so desperately ill—and turned away.

If there is any consolation at the moment, it's the encouraging responses I'm receiving as a result of my personal letter writing campaign. Noted specialists throughout the nation are inviting me to their facilities for consultation. And they're doing so based on my symptoms, as I described them. Even before meeting them, I detect a respect for what I have to say, an interest in my case and a sincere desire to help. From the responses I receive, I select and schedule an appointment with a rheumatologist in a nearby state.

Regardless of my body's determination not to cooperate, tomorrow we leave for our annual Cape Cod vacation. A July event I usually anticipate, counting the days until its arrival, this year is just the opposite. Inwardly lamenting not feeling well enough to approach our imminent holiday with my usual enthusiasm, the truth is, I don't—a truth that, if I can help it, no one else in my family will discover.

Even the most minimal packing I can get away with is difficult. I'm nauseated just looking down long enough to fold a tee shirt. The letters on its slogan are a blur. I feel like I'm trying to focus on them immediately after swimming underwater, before I've had a chance to blink out the excess liquid. Yet, when I touch my eyes, they feel dry. I'm dizzy, lightheaded and experiencing an intense headache. Touching the outside of my nose activates severe discomfort from the large, bleeding, internal ulcers.

A prominent, butterfly-shaped rash, characteristic of lupus, shades my face lavender-pink. At the moment, it is raised, with symmetrical bumps on both cheeks. My hair is thinning along the hairline, though thankfully nowhere near as rapidly as at the inception of the connective-tissue disease, when I lost handfuls daily. Round-the-clock I double over from waves of severe abdominal cramps, associated with electric-like chills occurring one minute on, one minute off. Throughout the day, I concertedly suppress the overwhelming urge to vomit.

My muscles and joints scream with pain only I can hear. Swollen legs and feet cause unsteadiness when I walk. My fingers and toes turn color from Raynoud's phenomenon. Suffocating panic jolts me out of my sleep, desperately gasping for air. Muscles jerk involuntarily and seizure-like vibrating is an everyday occurrence. I can't imagine that I'm not dying.

Is it any surprise vacation leaves a lot to be desired? From the day we arrive, I long for the week to go by fast. As much as I try to enjoy reliving Cape Cod memories of the past—long walks leaving our footprints on wet, squishy sandbars rippled by retreated waves, elaborate sandcastles constructed at the water's edge, beautiful sunsets that disappear into the ocean, sea gulls communicating in a dialogue all their own—it's not the same. Correction, I'm not the same.

Considering the fact that Tim and Stacey are vacationing with us, along with Storey's boyfriend, whose work schedule limits his visit to only a few days, my current health-related limitations are especially disconcerting. Though I want to do everything I can to make it special for all of them, I feel like I belong in a hospital. Somehow, I've got to camouflage this unnerving reality for the sake of everyone's vacation. "Please God, let me be the only one aware of how desperately ill I really am this week"

Momentarily distracting my thoughts from emphasis on myself, I nostalgically think back to how things have changed since we first purchased our timeshare vacation fourteen years ago. Stacey was six and Storey not quite two. With the largest outdoor pool on the Cape, an indoor pool, and the ocean at our doorstep, the girls took full advantage of the swim lessons they were enrolled in since the time they were only months old. To this day, the friends we met the year we bought, and have vacationed next door to ever since that time, marvel at how tiny Storey looked, petite for eighteen months as she was, diving into the huge pool.

Stacey immediately became friends with the girl next door. They were virtually inseparable, and comfortable accompanying each other's family to miniature golf, boat rides and out to restaurants.

After dinner, Eddie, Stacey, Storey and I would collect shells at the water's edge. Hand-in-hand with our daughters, we experienced family bonding at its best. Over the years, we accumulated irreplaceable memories of times none of us will ever forget. And the tradition goes on, with subtle, and sometimes not so subtle, changes. The girls still walk the beach—but they've found other hands to hold. Watching from a distance as they jump waves, laugh and run along the shoreline, hand-in-hand, with the boyfriends they've come to love, reality hits. We've done our part, the time is right and change is inevitable.

Swallowing the lump in my throat, I blink my misty eyes dry and, as I reach for Eddie's hand, say a silent prayer that the men in my daughters' lives will be as good to them as the gentleman walking beside me. Together we head back to our unit.

The week, in spite of its far-less-than-perfect weather and my debilitating symptoms, still manages to be fun. Fortunately, I'm able to camouflage my worst episodes from the kids. As luck would have it, on the day I feel the most nauseated, they decide to take off to a distant beach. To encourage this decision, which will afford the privacy I crave to lie in bed the entire day, without arousing suspicion, I prepare a picnic lunch for them. They see this as a thoughtful gesture on my part. Though it is intended to be, far stronger motivation is the maternal protection instinct that desperately drives me to shelter them from my pain.

By the time they return, hours later, my nausea is just beginning to subside. The strong urge to vomit has lessened. I prepare dinner with resurrected enthusiasm I rarely exhibit anymore, as I inquire about their day.

I'm inarguably more lethargic this vacation, content to stay in our unit writing and struggling to read the numbers corresponding to crossword clues. Occasionally Storey's boyfriend, who I adore and will always occupy a special place in my heart, and I attempt to solve a puzzle together. When we do, he often deciphers the numbers for me or, tactfully corrects the many situations when I misread the number of the corresponding clue.

On the one night we do venture out, a strong but tender arm draws me nearer as the concert hall darkens. The song Eddie selected twenty-five years ago for our wedding dance, "This Guy's in Love With You", brings a tear of happiness, a tear of irreplaceable memories, a tear of anticipated tomorrows, to my eye. As the male vocalist melodically bellows out the words, "Who looks at you the way I do?", I look into the same loving eyes that have reflected back at mine, after all these years, and answer the rhetorical question silently: "No one.

"As the end of our week approaches, it is without the usual regret I feel when vacation is almost over. Part of the reason I'm anxious to get back is to check the mail, hoping for more positive responses to my letter writing campaign.

chapter seventeen

Nationwide Medical Contacts

Picking up the week's mail from our rural delivery box, a hospital return address immediately catches my eye. Of the several responses I received, this one, in particular, outlining a well-researched diagnostic plan, appeals the most. It is written by a neurologist. According to him, based on the information I provided in my letter, in conjunction with the test results I forwarded, I clearly have central nervous system involvement. In consulting with a rheumatologist on staff at his facility, known for its success with lupus patients, it is suspected that the source of my neurological problems is the connective-tissue disease.

The doctors are confident that with my history of significant abnormal studies, there should be an identifiable answer. He invites me to the hospital, for admittance to the sleep study unit, which he directs. Additionally, he wants to repeat other neurological tests and scans. Unlike previous physicians who told me I'm not sick enough to be admitted, he warns me that this will require a week's stay. I almost can't believe what I'm reading. A physician is willing to take the risk and admit me based solely on information I've provided. How affirming,—not to mention potentially life-saving. And I want to jump at the opportunity.

Instead, since the hospital is three thousand miles away, and I already have an appointment, tomorrow, with a specialist located within three hours of my home, (one who responded prior to vacation), I resist the urge. I owe it to myself to keep this appointment, made with a rheumatologist described as "one of the best in the country", before considering the distant-but-tempting neurologist's invitation. Eddie and I agree that if the visit doesn't elucidate my condition to the point of an aggressive treatment plan, instituted immediately, I will be on the first plane out to the other facility.

A couple of weeks ago, in anticipation of this important appointment, I asked one of my specialist's for an introductory letter to bring along. The short paragraph I received in return summarized every normal test result I've had, stating that my neurological symptoms remain unexplained. Not one abnormal report was included. I became so angry reading it, I swear I could feel my blood seethe. I don't think it is asking too much of my doctors to at least document the facts objectively.

Reading the paragraph to Trixie, during one of her nightly phone calls I depend on, she comments, "It sounds like the physician who wrote that is making you out to be a hypochondriac"—Eddie's and my feelings, precisely. With slanted opinions such as this, is there any hope that I'll ever get diagnosed? Recognizing that the letter will do me more harm than good, I discard it.

Instead, I research my past medical reports, diligently recording every normal and abnormal finding I can locate since the lights' incident. Following is the chronological outline I created in place of the doctor's introductory paragraph.

CLINICAL FINDINGS
3-94 to present

Date	**Text/Scan/Exam**	**Result**
3 '94	C.A.T. Scan (head)	Negative*
4 '94	Neurologist's Exam	Inability to detect cold on hands, feet and forehead
4 '94	Ophthamologist's Exam	Hole in retina
4 '94	M.R.I. (head)	Normal
4 '94	Evoked Potential	Normal
4 '94	Neurologist's Exam	Cyanosis/toes Distal Hyperstesia to cold
5 '94	Neurology Work-Up	Positive: Nystagmus on Dix-Hallpike maneuvers with head turned to the left and right. Distal Hyperstesia to cold and pinprick over upper and lower extremities, bilaterally

* Later abnormal scan indicated that, in retrospect, ischemia noticed in the subsequent scan may have been present in the first one but obscured due to technical factors.

Date	Text/Scan/Exam	Result
5 '94	M.R.I. (head)	Normal
6 '94	Spinal Tap	Normal
6 '94	S.P.E.C.T. Scan	Abnormal: Hypoperfusion in left temporal cortex attributable to Lupus Cerebritis/ Vasculitis
7 '94	Rheumatologist's Exam	Slurred speech
7 '94	Echocardiogram	Small Mitral Valve Prolapse. Mildy/ Moderately Depressed left Ventricular Systolic Function
8 '94	Neurologist's Exam	Unexplained urinary incontinence
8 '94	Rheumatologist's Exam	Drooling, slurred speech
10 '94	Pet Scan	Normal
10 '94	Ambulatory E.E.G.	Abnormal: Bi-temporal slowing with sharp features predominant in left temporal area
11 '94	Rheumatology Work-Up	Positive Ana (1:160) Speckled Pattern. Malar Rash, Raynouds ???Vasculitis
11 '84	C.A.T. Scan (head)	Ischemia, left side
12 '94	Split Screen E.E.G.	Abnormal: Temporal Dysrhythmia
2 '95	Neurological Work-Up	Positive, R. Eye Negative, L. Eye
	Schrimer's Test:	White Count: 4,000 Slightly Elevated Sed Rate, Positive Thyroid Antibodies
4 '95	Lip Biopsy	Negative

Date	Text/Scan/Exam	Result
5 '95	Sleep Study	Abnormal: 46 awakenings and 125 arousals within 4 hours. According to report, 25 arousals per hour is markedly elevated
7 '95	Rheumatologist's Exam	Tender, swollen right knee with synovial thickening
8 '95	Neurologist's Exam	Fuzzy optic discs, brisk upper extremities
10 '95	Fluorescein Angiogram	DECREASED blood flow to optic nerve
2 '96	Cardiologist's Exam	Abdominal bruit. ? Abdominal aortic aneurysm possibly due to vasculitis
3 '96	Arteriograms (Head and Intestines)	Abdominal spasms upon insertion, otherwise normal study. Tachycardia evidenced at conclusion.
4 '96	Ophthamologist's Exam	Optic nerves cupped pale inferiorly, suggests decreased perfusion

Scenery flies by, not all of it pretty, as our train approaches the big city. Opting for public transportation, many visitors from our area agree it is the most practical way of accessing the city. Besides, it's an education in itself.

Looking around, we're surrounded by faceless commuters hidden behind identical editions of open newspapers. Others, who arrived too late to find a seat on this rush hour express, stand precariously in any nook and cranny available. Every time the train's brakes are applied, so are theirs'.

Too interested in observing those around me to concentrate on my crossword, I let it drop to my feet. Instead, my mind is occupied creating scenarios as to why various individuals travel, most of them undoubtedly on a regular basis, to this incredible city I seldom visit. Inarguably, the lady in the suit, clutching a burgundy leather portfolio and cardboard cup of what I assume is coffee, is a career woman.

Then there's the guy in his early twenties, dressed in a white tee shirt, cut off jeans and a faded baseball cap, the kind you pay extra for because of the comfy, weathered, broken-in look. A college student on summer break, en route to visit a friend, perhaps?

Awkwardly meeting the gaze of a male commuter standing directly opposite my seat, I'm uncomfortable and quickly avert my eyes. A middle-aged man, whose professional attire begs for an iron, squishes more of himself into the remaining seat availability than there is room for, cramming me up against the cool metal wall of my window seat.

There's an unmistakable impersonalness reflected in the lack of interaction among commuters. They share the same train, yet nothing of themselves. No one talks to their seat mate, many stare straight ahead, there are few smiles. Uncomfortable in this unfriendly environment, I'm anxious for the ride to end.

Pulling into the station, Eddie and I let the rushing horde of people race by our seat. We can wait the extra few minutes. As the variety of commuters pass us by, I ask myself if any of them could possibly have as much riding on their visit, as I do on mine. The unspoken answer to my question unnerves me.

I guess I've lived in a rural town too long to develop a full appreciation for the city. Clinging to my seat for dear life, my hands feel sweaty against the soft vinyl upholstery. The look I shoot Eddie doesn't require verbalization. He accurately assesses my evaluation of our cabbie's driving. The rolled eyes he gives in return signal that he concurs. With a tightening knot of anxiety, as we weave in and out of traffic much faster than we should, barely beat traffic lights, and place unsuspecting pedestrians in danger, it is a relief to reach the doctor's office without casualty.

Dr. Crandall's closet-like exam room is a claustrophobic's nightmare. Fortunately, neither Eddie nor I are afflicted with this self-limiting phenomenon. In a room smaller than many bathrooms I've seen is a table, a sink that you barely clear closing the door, and a small oval wall mirror. Just as I note there isn't even a stool for the doctor, he enters the room and remains standing, out of necessity.

Not two feet away from me, due to the forced proximity determined by the parameters of the room, I look into this man's eyes, mentally trying to assess his ability as a physician. Is he as accomplished as his reputation claims? Haven't I already seen some of the best that major medical centers have to offer? Will he, too, turn me away? Or can he read the indisguisable desperation in my eyes, the look that says this person may be dying—and I'd better act quickly.

With these unspoken questions left temporarily unanswered in my mind, I shake Dr. Crandall's outstretched hand. Following introductory ice-breaker comments that provide insight into his outwardly pleasant personality, we get right down to business. As I sequentially detail the history of this illness, he listens intently. The nature of his questions reflect connections he's making in his own mind—connections neither I nor the majority of other physicians I've seen, considered. And I'm encouraged.

His exam is similar to the rheumatological work-ups I've had in the past except the observations he shares, are many. He notes dry eyes, mouth, and nose, bleeding nasal ulcers, Raynoud's phenomenon, a malar rash across the cheeks and painful muscles and joints. Concluding the physical, he gathers my medical records and heads toward his office, asking Eddie and I to join him once I've gotten dressed. Apprehensively, we follow.

Up until now, I don't know what he's thinking—but I do know he's identified definite abnormalities. When he begins his analysis of my condition, however, seated behind a desk half covered with a collection of miniature antique cars I assume were donated by grateful patients, his first few words prepare me for letdown. "Certainly you've had connective-tissue disease long enough to realize how painful it can be". Here it comes. He's going to tell me that, like other afflicted patients, I've no choice but to learn to live with it. And like so many other physicians, he'll miss the point—that it's not the pain, but the life-threatening potential of my particular case, that demands treatment—NOW. But miraculously, he doesn't repeat the words of denial I've come to dread. Instead, he continues explaining, "If your connective-tissue involvement was limited to joint and muscle pain, as much as I'd feel for you, it wouldn't be life-threatening. With Central Nervous System involvement", which according to him is indisputable in my case, "immediate and aggressive intervention is imperative."

To further demonstrate the urgency involved, he describes a patient currently hospitalized with the same condition. "Though intelligent to the point that she has The Gettysburg Address, The Preamble to The Constitution and Emily Dickinson poetry committed to memory, she can't recall that she's married." An unnerving chill passes through me at the realization that my deepest fears, shared in desperate, undisclosed letters to my family, were not unfounded.

Even without hearing the regiment of treatment he's about to recommend, I'm overwhelmed with what I've just learned. My emotions vacillate from indescribable gratitude to this physician for unlocking this medical mystery, to unnerving fear that a leading expert in the field has confirmed that my physical state is every bit as grave as I've assumed all along. Listening with indistractable attentiveness, he explains, "The only logical course of action is pulse chemotherapy, administered monthly, on an out-patient basis at your local hospital". No sooner are the words out of his mouth, before my mind transports me back to a doctor's appointment two years ago, when I begged one of my physicians to institute aggressive chemotherapy. Convinced at the time that the connective-tissue disease was attacking my entire nervous system, I researched treatment and learned that this was the procedure of choice. The physician I approached told me, "I have no proof a vascular process is attacking your nervous system, and, consequently, can't justify a regiment that is not without considerable risk".

When I asked how vascular neurological involvement is proven, she replied, "By brain biopsy. However, it is next to impossible to detect even then because it requires such a precise sample". Now, two agonizing years later, one of the top specialists in the country is telling me I can't start aggressive treatment soon enough. The irony of the moment is only surpassed by my frustration with previous medical interaction.

Continuing, Dr. Crandall explains, "From the disease's inception twelve years ago, you've exhibited signs of Central Nervous System involvement—but to a much lesser degree. The cascading lights' episode triggered more serious symptoms such as the blurry vision, involuntary muscle jerking, disassociation, numbness, pins-and-needles, brisk reflexes, urinary incontinence, tingling and nausea."

Once again, my mind flashes back, this time to the many incidents in which neurologists looked at me like I was some kind of a fool when I described numbness on both sides of my body. Repeatedly, I was told that was impossible. Didn't it ever occur to them that a connective-tissue disease, attacking the nervous system, could produce symptoms bi-laterally? If not, I suggest they go back to school and read up on this life-threatening condition!

My silent tirade is interrupted with Dr. Crandall's unmistakable look of concern, followed up by, "Do you have any questions?". Almost too overwhelmed to think, the only question that comes to mind is, "When will treatment begin?". "As soon as I can get in touch with Dr. Michaels to recommend a dosage." I know Eddie just asked him something, also, but for the life of me, I can't remember what, I'm so pre-occupied. With a knowing, compassionate look in my direction, one that says when all this sinks in you'll have plenty of questions, he adds, "Feel free to call me if anything else comes up". Before I realize it, we're shaking hands once more with the physician who just may be responsible for saving my life—or, at least trying. Somehow, even the sincere thank-you I offer is inadequate.

Over lunch, Eddie and I engage in conversation consumed by our reactions to the rheumatologist's diagnosis and proposed course of action. My husband comments honestly, "My feelings are mixed. While grateful that a physician, whose opinion in the rheumatological field is considered inarguable, has conclusively identified the problem, I'm frightened by its serious connotations." I agree. The only thing scarier than the treatment he prescribed is where I was before this appointment—the only one aware of how desperately I needed aggressive and immediate medical intervention with potent drugs. My long, painful search has ended. After two and a half years of intolerable, bizarre symptoms, I now have an explanation and direction, which is all I sought right along. Finally, a competent specialist heard me and has a plan.

Or so I thought! A few days later, the specialist calls. After reconsideration, he decides not to bring in the "heavy artillery" yet. Instead, he recommends a much less potent drug, first. It's his hope that this medication will eliminate the need for the other. No sooner than I hang up the phone with him, it rings again. It's Dr. Michaels.

Apparently he and Dr. Crandall had a detailed conversation about my case. According to him, the later drug proposed is a male hormone proven helpful in decreasing some lupus symptoms. Call me vain, but an image of growing a beard materializes in my head. Until now, as much as this disease has robbed me of my being, my femininity is still intact—and I'd like to keep it that way.

I question Dr. Michaels regarding whether I would take on the male characteristics I envision. His honest, but affirmative answer, is depressing. Sensing my discouragement, he quickly follows his answer up with reality: "It beats death." Inarguably, he's right. But, once again, I feel negatively controlled by the ramifications of this impossible disease. I know I'm expected to sit back and agree, but it's not that easy. I guess the only way to put it in perspective for a male physician would be to ask how he would feel if advised to take an experimental medication which would make him grow large breasts.

Thinking better of sharing this analogy, instead I ask him if it is expected to address the neurological symptoms associated with this disease: the nausea, dizziness, visual disturbance, doubling over cramping and body-wrenching chills. His response stresses its success with muscle and joint pain, rather than neurological symptoms. That's all the convincing I need to decide against the drug. I've lived with muscle and joint pain for the twelve years I've had this disease. I don't see it as life-threatening, just painful—certainly not worth a drug with such unfeminine side affects, as far as I'm concerned.

At the same time, he warns me that the dosage of chemotherapy the specialist is considering is high enough to have residual lethal side affects. I'm completely blown away by this revelation! At my recent visit, I had no idea we were discussing such a massive dose. Another physician I spoke to last week assured me that chemotherapy used for lupus patients is far less potent than that used for Cancer patients, consequently void of the side affects of hair loss and excessive nausea. But that's not what I'm hearing now—and Dr. Michaels verified the dosage with Dr. Crandall just this morning. I'm sure his information is more updated and accurate than mine.

Questioning him further, I explain I was unaware of the potency of the chemotherapy originally suggested. The first to admit he's not a Cancer specialist, Dr. Michaels offers to consult one. Undoubtedly, an oncologist who, in his practice prescribes high doses of this medication, will have more specific information regarding its dangers.

His research proves discouraging. The treatment considered is every bit as ominous as he'd intimated. Desperate and confused, I ask one of the few physicians I trust, "What would you do?". Hesitating, he acknowledges, "It's a tough call and in the end, it's your decision—one that I will support, either way." Reluctantly, I request that he schedule the chemotherapy. Moments later I retract that decision, reflecting the current confusion of my mind. One thing I AM sure of, this is not the time to act impulsively. Electing a treatment with such serious ramifications requires far more thought.

The tears start to fall before I hang up the phone. At this time last week, I was so relieved. I finally had a diagnosis and what I looked at as a manageable treatment plan. I was anxious for it to begin. Unaware of the risks, my main focus was getting help for the unendurable neurological symptoms. Just last night, as I intentionally prevented myself from falling asleep on my back, fearful that I'd awaken with the suffocating sensation this position encourages, I thought optimistically that once the new treatment begins, this may no longer be a threat—and now this!

Unintentional as it may be, I feel like my emotions have been chewed up and spit back out at me by a medical profession oblivious to what all this is doing to my sanity. From day to day, I don't know what doctor to believe, whether abnormal test results will be respected or, as in the past, discredited by skeptical physicians, if a treatment plan I come to terms with one day will suddenly be revoked the next, or what my tenuously uncertain future has in store for me. Granted, my case may not be clear-cut, but this indecisiveness is driving me crazy.

Dear Stacey:

As much as I've tried to prepare you, how does a mom prepare her daughter for a time like this? Whenever I heard your cheerful voice, (and wishful thinking), on the other end of the phone, trying to convince yourself as much as me, "I just know you're getting better!", I thought, "No, honey, that's not the case; unfortunately, I'm getting worse." Understandably, that's not what you wanted to hear—or I wanted to say.

Until now, I thought only eyes cried, but believe me there are tears in my heart as well. You have no idea how much your daily calls have meant to me. I couldn't have faced this scary time without them. Beyond a doubt, the love, closeness and tenderness at the root of our relationship came through in your kind actions. I put so much, (and I know you did, too), into that hug at the bus terminal—because I was afraid I wouldn't get another chance. I tried to squeeze hard enough to give you love to last a lifetime. No one has any guarantees, but having been sick for so many years, I approached motherhood with the idea that I would do everything possible with, and for, my children, thinking that if I lived a long time, they'd have a wonderful life; on the other hand, if I didn't, they would have tons of special times to remember. I hope I accomplished this, honey, because I tried so hard.

Beyond a doubt, the strategy encouraged such a close and special bond between us—one that only we can know. The experiences we've shared in the past, and how you feel about them, are memories no one can take from you. NEVER forget that. People live together a lifetime and don't know the amount of love we're blessed with. The truth is, I feel so very sick—and so scared. And, I'm angry. I've asked myself over and over tonight why women who abuse their children and hate their husbands walk around in perfect health, when someone who loves her family more than words can express, lives in fear of losing that privilege.

I'm worried about you, hon. Because I know you, I know the trauma you're experiencing like no one else can. Believe me, if I had any control, I'd put an end to this nightmare, but we both know I don't. No matter what my future holds, please, please don't let it affect your plans, hopes and dreams. Know my sincere wish is that you fulfill each and every one of them.

As difficult as these times are, you've got to be strong and pull together with dad and Storey, for the sake of our family. There is so much love there—and if ever you guys needed it to fall back on, it's now.

Finally, if I ever reach a point where I can no longer communicate with you, rest assured we'll still be connected in our hearts. When you have difficult decisions to make, or doubts as to what to do, consider "If I could ask mom's opinion, what would she say?". The love we share will guide you in your actions.

I can't see through my tears to write anymore but you know how I feel. You occupy a special place in my heart that's reserved only for you—and always will.

Love,
Mom

And following a few hours time out to compose myself...

Dear Storey:

My perceptive and supportive, not-so-little daughter, how would I have gotten through this incredibly difficult time without you? Did I lean on you too hard? If I did, I apologize but, honey, I needed you so badly. You'll never know how much your support helped. Through adverse conditions, our hearts touched in an indescribable way—a way only you and I know.

Your words of comfort were not only reassuring, but realistic. I feel as though I shed a zillion tears on your little shoulders—but I'm so glad they were there. The tears you couldn't see, but undoubtedly sensed, were the ones in my heart. I'm absolutely tormented. It was like I couldn't hug you enough, Storey. Never forget those hugs and their intensity, because they contained all my love for you—love I want you to have forever.

It goes without saying that if I could go back in time to healthier days, I would. But, Storey, we both know better. God knows, I've wracked my brain trying to resolve this nightmare. Instead, I'm forced to sit back and let whatever happens, happen. I don't need to tell you what a frightening position I'm in. You've lived it right along side of me. You understand it in a way no one else does, and I love you for that, (and a lot of other reasons!)

By now you know the kinds of things I want for you in life. And I know the kinds of things you want for you. Though you'll always be an individual, in many ways,. we're on the same wavelength.

You're blessed with intellect beyond your years. Use it to make good decisions, as I know you will. If, at anytime you're faced with a dilemma not easily solved, and my physical state is not conducive to offering guidance, fall back on past advice and, if you elect to, adapt it to the current situation.

I know this is an awful position for a teenager to be in, and that it's not fair. You deserve the security of knowing your mom is available to you. I'm sick at heart at the thought that this stability is threatened. You deserve so much more.

Regardless of any physical disability or mental impairment this condition may generate in future years, and/or the distortion of my original role of the mother you knew, know that wherever you are in life, a part of me will always be with you. I love you and will forever. Adopting you was one of the best decisions of my life!

Love,
Mom

The red telephone message button is lit and blinking incessantly, its unexpected and ominous presence sending chills of concern up and down my spine, as we return to our hotel room. Only Stacey and Storey know the location of our spur-of-the-moment, weekend getaway—and neither would call unless it were an emergency.

The phone shaking in my hand, it's a struggle to find the coordination necessary to punch in "0" and connect with the front desk. By the time I succeed, my heart is racing and my legs feel like rubber. Sweating profusely during the eternity it seems to take for the person on the other end to locate the message, my eyes close while my lips automatically tense into a tight line as the operator repeats words I dread hearing: "Call Stacey as soon as possible." The extra, sixth sense all mothers possess warns me it isn't good.

My lungs feel ready to burst as I unintentionally hold my breath, while Eddie finishes dialing her number. The coward in me leaves the responsibility of initial contact to him. Not surprisingly, Stacey answers on the first ring, undoubtedly sitting next to the phone awaiting our return call. Desperately, I try to read Eddie's eyes for some sign. At first, they protectively avert mine. But seconds later they focus on me, intensely, open wider than normal in undisguised concern. "Honey, try to calm down. Don't let yourself jump to conclusions until you have the benefit of test results. The doctors are just trying to be thorough in using a process of elimination approach", he soothes long-distance. But I'm unconvinced by what are meant to be reassuring words. Unlike Stacey, I can see his worried, brow-creased expression—he's scared. And why is he talking to her about doctors and test results? What could possibly be wrong?

Whether I'm prepared to face what's happening or not, my questions are about to be answered when, at Stacey's request, he hands the phone to me. Bursting into tears at the sound of my voice, I can only make out a few words. Unfortunately, they include "tumor" and "brain". That's all I need to hear to dissolve into tears myself. Sobbing silently, but uncontrollably, I pray "Please, God, not one of my children. I'm ready to bargain, big-time. I'll take anything I have coming my way but please let Stacey be healthy." To her, I speak as calmly as possible, though unsuccessful is disguising the tears in my voice.

Eventually, she calms down enough to communicate that she'd seen an ear, nose and throat specialist today for a continual popping, crackling sensation in her ear. Completely surprising her, a hearing test on the affected ear revealed significant auditory loss. Frighteningly, only through lip-reading could she recognize that the technician was inquiring, "Can't you hear me?". To this point, she was unaware of a hearing loss. Yet in reality, her hearing decreased by more than 50%.

Tearfully, she informs me that her doctor ordered a stat M.R.I. of her head, suspecting a tumor. As a fourth year nursing student, she realizes the immediacy of scheduling a test is directly proportionate to a physician's concern regarding the gravity of a patient's condition. As a seasoned patient, I know that, too. However, with her panicky state subsiding minimally, I'm able to discern that the type of tumor suspected is not on the brain but near the ear. It is the close proximity to the brain that would require both an ear, nose and throat surgeon and a neuro-surgeon for removal. "Stacey, what you're telling me is significantly different than a brain tumor", I allow my mind to think out loud, undisguised relief in my voice. "But, mom, they said I'd need a neuro-surgeon!", she counters emphatically.

Understanding the situation a little better by this point, I pull myself together and automatically revert into the reassuring mom mode. "Honey, I had a neuro-surgeon operate on my lumbar disk, as a precaution, due to the delicate area. And I didn't have a brain tumor. I know it's scary to consider the need for a neuro-surgeon but, trust me, these specialists do many other types of surgery, as well." "But, Mom, I'm so scared! I failed the hearing test so drastically. Before I walked into the office I didn't even realize I had a hearing loss. The results shocked my physician, too. As a matter-of-fact, she wasn't even going to conduct a hearing test because I told her I hadn't noticed any loss. It was an afterthought, as I was on my way out the door, that she decided to do a precautionary one. And I'm glad she did! It's always better to diagnose at as early a stage as possible", she says as the benefit of her nurse's training kicks in. Unfortunately, there is a negative side to knowing too much. Ironically, she just began her rotation on Pediatric Oncology today and worries that if a tumor is found, it could be cancerous. Talk about poor timing for the start of that rotation!

She's so scared, my inclination is to jump in the car and be with her. Eddie helps put things in perspective. She's twelve hours away. We wouldn't arrive before the M.R.I. was conducted, anyway. Tim is with her and will be by her side during the scan. A more realistic approach is to leave for home. We will arrive in Connecticut during her M.R.I. and know the results within minutes of getting home. If a surgical procedure is required, we will head straight to Syracuse. It is this kind of logic that Eddie uses that makes us compatible, by balancing it with my more emotional and impulsive reactions.

Understanding Eddie's point, while he packs up our things I talk to the doctor, who explains the immediacy of the scan is due to the fact that if a tumor does exist, the sooner it is addressed, the better her chances of preventing further hearing loss. Even with the specialist's efforts to reassure me, I hang up the phone numb.

Her situation served as a wake-up call for me. With a sheepish expression I hide from others, I reflect on how just a few hours earlier, as I dried my hair, I wrapped the towel in a single layer around my head, trying to envision just how unflattering it will be if I lose my hair, should chemotherapy and/or radiation, treatment options under consideration, be necessary. How vain! It reminds me of when, as a teenager, my friend, (later-turned-sister-in-law), and I, the week before getting braces, used aluminum foil to try to simulate what we'd look like ahead of time. That's the interesting thing about writing. Though everybody does dumb things from time to time, writers share these experiences with others—and I think that's healthy. Not only do they come to terms with the fact that they're not expected to be perfect, they learn it's okay to admit to their imperfections—even laugh at them, while at the same time entertaining others.

Fumbling with the key, I awkwardly unlock the door as quickly as possible, reacting to the ringing phone I hear faintly from the porch. Running to the closest telephone, I'm greeted by a cheerful and relaxed Stacey on the other end. She doesn't have to tell me the outcome of her test. I'm already silently thanking God for the obvious answer, verified by the undisguised relief in her voice. There is no tumor. As it turns out, when the technician re-checked her hearing following the normal scan, it was perfect. Sheepishly, she admits to our daughter that the sound wasn't turned on in the testing booth during the original test. Collapsing into a nearby chair, my mind at ease, it occurs to me that whoever believes the responsibilities of being a parent, and the concerns associated with that role, end as the child becomes an adult is grossly dissolutioned—at least in my book. My grown children will always remain a priority in my life, and can call on me at anytime. That's what love is all about.

Bundled in a tee shirt, a turtleneck, two flannel shirts, a pullover sweater, a jacket, corduroy pants, woolen ski socks and lined boots, I convulse with chills. A neurologist in closer proximity to my home, than the majority I've been seeing lately, opens the door to the exam room, too angry to notice—or care. Omitting any greeting, he bluntly informs me, "Your university specialist never called me. Besides, I don't have time in my day to spend on the phone discussing your case. If he wants to communicate with me, tell him to write me a letter". My eyes smart with stinging tears I fight to hold back.

The call he dismisses so nonchalantly is of optimal importance to me—and he knows it. I told him immediately following my appointment with a university specialist, a month ago, that the doctor wanted to speak to him about collectively formulating a treatment plan. Struggling to keep my quivering voice steady, I ask, "Did you try to contact him?". With fire in his eyes, he raises his voice, "I have no intention of calling him!". Further enraged, he continues, "And I'm certainly not going to agree to a treatment plan to radiate your brain, as your note informed me he suggested. It's a death sentence. Let him do it."

Unable to hold back the flood gates any longer, rivers stream down my cheeks as I barely manage to get out, "Won't I die if the strokes remain untreated?". His answer, "Probably", is automatic and void of any compassion. As he continues, I can't believe the things I'm hearing. "Maybe you should find another doctor. Nobody wants your case." "But I have so many abnormal findings, including every brain test", I counter. "That's the problem. You have so much going on, no doctor wants to risk treating you—including me."

At the word "risk", MALPRACTICE flashes across my brain, every doctor's fear—a sad commentary on medicine in the 1990s. That's why he doesn't want to commit to a treatment plan associated with serious and potentially lethal side affects. Yet, if this isn't attacked pro-actively, I could die anyway. I think the decision to take risks should be the patient's, even if it means signing a paper absolving the doctor of blame. It's my body—and my life. How dare someone else tell me I can't try everything possible to save it? Would his response be the same if it was HIS wife and the mother of HIS children?

The visit quickly goes from bad to worse. He holds up a list of times saying, "Do you know what my day is like? I start out at six o'clock in the morning and"...I don't give him a chance to finish, interjecting "Doctor, do you know what MY day is like?" "I'm sure it's miserable", he concedes. Continuing, I tell him I think it's pathetic that in an entire month medical professionals were too "busy" to find time to touch base on such a serious case.

I verbalize the obvious. "I'm not a doctor. I'm not qualified to treat myself. Yet, I feel frustrated because those who are, won't. Eddie and I are so desperate, we're thinking of conducting a Med-Line search", I admit. "Maybe you should", comes the unfeeling response.

In a last ditch effort to seek his cooperation, and procure the medical intervention my serious symptoms blatantly indicate, I show him an article I cut out of this week's newspaper. It describes the rare and potentially deadly illness, Central Nervous System vasculitis, in which the patient's immune system reacts against its own blood vessels, resulting in multiple strokes. It denotes a patient whose symptoms parallel many of mine. In addition to memory and visual problems, she has a defective temperature control mechanism. Interestingly, a nurse in town saw it and commented that it sounded like me. The treatment, which has been effective in her case, includes high dose steroids and chemotherapy.

The article makes no effort to minimize the potentially lethal affects of such therapy; on the other hand, it focuses on the deadly outcome if the destructive vascular process isn't arrested. "I'd need more proof than I've seen, that you have vasculitis", he says, completely discounting the fact that a previous S.P.E.C.T. scan reported it. "And that's often next to impossible to get. Besides, with the treatment recommended in the article, you'll lose all your hair", he points out using a different psychology to discourage me. Though I care about my appearance, at the moment, I have far more serious concerns on my mind—like attending our daughters' weddings, sharing retirement years with Eddie, and eventually having grandchildren to read to.

At the conclusion of one of the most horrendous doctors' appointments I can recall, (and that's a pretty strong statement from someone who has been emotionally mistreated by so many physicians), I leave in sobbing tears, unable to remain in the waiting room while the person I came with has her physical. Once again, I feel like the patient no doctor wants—and with good reason!

chapter eighteen

Up, Up and Away

The turmoil of indecision viciously eats away at my mind, like a parasite devouring its host. Obsessed by the all-consuming fear of potential lethal repercussions, from massive chemotherapy, my brain is in overdrive searching for a less ominous solution. One alternative that repeatedly surfaces throughout this mind-boggling process is the invitation I received the day before my appointment with Dr. Crandall—the one from a neurologist detailing a very specific, and by-the-day more tempting diagnostic approach. Unable to dismiss the logic behind such a comprehensive plan, I realize there's no decision to be made. I've got to go for it.

Eddie totally supports the consultation. The problem is that I will have to travel by myself. Though able to accompany me on the other, less-distant, out-of-state appointments, this facility is three thousand miles away, too long an absence for a sole bread winner who just started a new assignment. As a result, this individual who never even lived away at college, or vacationed by herself, for that matter, is about to embark on cross-country travel, for a week, to face revelations thus far unknown. Reluctant as she is for this solo venture, it's a priority.

As the day of my flight quickly approaches, part of me almost can't believe I'm actually going through with it. Nor can Trixie, who expects me to back out last minute. Yet at 5:30 Sunday morning, while the rest of the state sleeps, I kiss Eddie good-bye before entering the turnstile, obeying the sign warning "Only ticket holding passengers beyond this point"—and reality hits.

Walking down the corridor juggling luggage far too heavy for me to comfortably carry, I feel so alone. And scared. A lot could happen to me before I see Eddie again next week, and probably will. More importantly, I may learn a lot—perhaps more than I'm ready to hear. With that unsettling thought manifesting in a rapidly developing cramp in the pit of my stomach, I walk through the security arch without setting off any buzzers, re-claim my purse from the conveyor, and board the plane.

Sitting by a window struggling to cram my carry-on bag under the seat in front of me, the pressurized chamber starts to affect my ears. Chewing gum to counteract the dull ache, I attempt to distract myself by observing the other passengers. People attired in business suits place briefcases in overhead carriers, while mothers give bottles of juice to crying infants. Children carrying stuffed Shammu's excitedly ramble on about their perspective trips to Sea World, where they will get to meet him in person. So many people—so varied the destinations.

Families obviously on vacations, excitedly planning their day-by-day, fun-packed agendas, revive memories of family adventures we've taken. Other travelers, visibly nervous, reference recent devastating air disasters, making it known the only reason they're flying is because it's the quickest method of transportation. Amid excitement, I see routine—and even sadness in some passengers aboard our flight. As the seat belt sign lights, I dutifully buckle up, placing my magazines and book on the empty seat next to me. But as we lift off, I can't concentrate on reading—my mind is too pre-occupied with what's ahead of me this week.

The list of specialists I'm scheduled to see seems overwhelming. Reviewing the no-time-to-breathe agenda the hospital forwarded, it is reminiscent of what a freshman receives when he first arrives on campus. Also included in the packet is an M.M.P.I., (Minnesota Multi-Phasic Personality Index), which consists of over five hundred subjective and ambiguous questions. Supposedly, based on the way a respondent answers these questions, a measure of his mental health status is derived. Among other things, it helps identify whether a patient is organically or psychologically ill. Here we go again!

If there's one reality I've discovered as a result of this illness, it's that difficult-to-diagnose cases, particularly those of women, invariably include a psychological profile. When conducted in conjunction with a battery of physical evaluations, such as this schedule incorporates, it's far more acceptable to me. The M.M.P.I. is more a nuisance than a concern. I'm physically ill and I'm confident my responses will corroborate that. However, the small print questions corresponding to hundreds of miniscule circle choices on the answer sheet grid are a nightmare for someone with blurry vision.

Aside from the logistics of completing that form, the neuro-psychologist who ordered it is the physician whose opinion I'm most interested in. The four hour block of time he's scheduled to see me includes far more than interpretation of the M.M.P.I. I'm to bring, completed, to the visit. In addition, he will conduct a series of exercises intended to evaluate long and short term memory, cognitive thinking, mathematical aptitude, sequential relationships, puzzle solving, reading comprehension, the ability to copy simple drawings, identify missing pieces on familiar items and, through these and numerous other checkpoints, diagnose any residual damage to the brain. In light of recent memory and speech changes I've noticed on my own, including unintentional reversal of categories and difficulty with word retrieval, I'm looking to him for answers to questions I've only begun to ask myself—but intend to share when we meet.

Having studied the filled-to-capacity schedule in detail, I'm optimistic this week will prove meaningful and well worth the distance I've traveled to make it happen. I guess I'm about to find out as the seat belt sign lights up and the plane lands safely at our destination.

Locating my shuttle, I head to the hospital-subsidized condo I reserved for the week. As fully equipped and pretty as it is, once registered, the only thing I see is the bed. I'm exhausted. The trip drained me physically. My muscles ache from the flight, I'm overdue for my headache medication, and despite dry temperatures in the nineties, which make this a popular vacation choice, I'm freezing. I order a room service cheeseburger, telephone Eddie and the girls, take a hot bath and am in bed by 7:30 p.m., which is really 10:30 p.m. by Eastern Daylight Time, the schedule my body is still on. Not surprisingly, I'm up by 3:30 a.m. I've had my night's sleep.

Monday morning initiates a week long medical marathon beyond my furthest dreams of realistic. I see more doctors, complete more forms and undergo more tests, scans, exams and interviews than I thought humanly possible in such a consolidated period. The scheduling is so tight, I find it difficult to get from one appointment to the next on time—and often don't. Breaks for meals are non-existent. On the rare occasion I do get one, it is invariably a non-nutritional snack on the fly.

I undergo an M.R.I. of the brain, an Electroencephalogram, E.M.G.s, an overnight sleep study, four hours of psychological and cognitive testing, a tilt table test, and extensive blood work. I see neurologists, rheumatologists, neuro-psychologists, ophthalmologists, neuro-ophthalmologists and neuro-muscular specialists, each of whom document detailed histories based on interviews slanted toward their piece of the puzzle.

Though I remain in daily contact with my family and friends, I'm alone, miles away from the hugs I crave, when I hear the disconcerting, but not surprising results. Every brain-related test and/or scan came out abnormal. The damage to my eyesight is permanent, resulting from the initial stroke, which, indisputably occurred when I saw lights. The original brain attack, along with five other ischemic strokes, is clearly evidenced on the M.R.I. Though I've had far more, only the larger ones get picked up on the scan.

My left eye and pupil measured larger than the right. Brain damage registered in several areas, corroborating, by location of the infarct, my complaint of switching categories and mis-using words, a form of aphasia often associated with strokes. Additionally, I've lost strength and dexterity in my dominant right hand. I demonstrate difficulty with number sequence and long term recall, inconsistent with that of a college graduate. Further, my E.M.G.s indicate generalized muscle weakness suggestive of the need for follow-up evaluation at a Muscular Dystrophy Clinic.

Understandably overwhelmed as the coordinating physician delivers all these serious findings at once, at the same time I'm grateful to get some answers, ominous though they may be. What I find mind-boggling is his assertion, "The important thing for you to hear is that the problem is organic", writing the word and underlining it for emphasis. Now tell me something I don't know! This man who just confirmed I sustained brain damage, with the potential for more should another episode occur, not to mention the potential for Muscular Dystrophy, is more concerned that I realize my physicians finally believe me, than with my reaction to the alarming medical facts uncovered.

Anger surging through my veins, while I simultaneously begin to tremble out of fear over my unnerving health status, I want to scream: "What do you think I've been trying to tell you guys for the past few years—while one doctor after another refused to hear me?". Instead, I vaguely register what he's saying, as he continues, "Not only are you organically ill, you're one of these people who, much to your own detriment, downplays both pain and illness. You don't ask for, or recognize the need for help soon enough".

I'm beyond angry; I'm livid. I had to travel three thousand miles for a diagnosis I not only suspected, but repeatedly questioned—one that local specialists were given ample opportunity to confirm.

Nothing short of inexcusable, the pathetic reality is that a stroke victim, fighting desperately for her life, was left to independently cope with severe residual symptoms because physicians refused to believe her.

Not one, but eleven* neurologists, all of whom were trained to recognize the stroke signs I exhibited, including dizziness, nausea, severe headache, blurry vision and slurred speech, prematurely dismissed my condition as psychological. With few exceptions, the more diligently I persisted in my pursuit of potentially life-saving treatment, the more adamantly I was rejected by the medical community. Experiencing more-terrifying-by-the-day, inexplicable symptoms, worse case scenarios consumed my thinking, flashing pessimistic scenes across the movie screen in my head. These daytime nightmares resulted in heart-wrenching letters to my family—trying to prepare them, and myself, for an uncertain future, filled with ominous undertones.

I now know that, as a confirmed multiple stroke patient, vascular involvement associated with the connective-tissue disease is responsible for this condition. In reality, my life was in jeopardy from the day I first sought medical attention—and still is. The potential for repeated, and even more serious attacks, is undeniable. The majority of my residual symptoms are permanent, resulting from the March 1994 stroke.

According to a representative I recently spoke to from The American Heart Association, I should have been hospitalized immediately on a stroke watch. Instead, I was told to see a Psychiatrist. If hospitalized, I would've been given therapy to address the physical changes incurred by this devastating brain attack. Additionally, the aphasia would have been addressed through speech therapy. Blood thinners would have been prescribed and untold heartache avoided just knowing a logical explanation existed for my overnight transformation into a person I no longer recognized.

Though I can't speak for other grossly mis-diagnosed patients, I, for one, refuse to complacently accept what occurred. I intend to do everything in my power to assure another patient doesn't unnecessarily live the hell I've been through. Writing this book is a first step toward public awareness. Should I end up dying from this condition, it won't be a wasted death—I'll have exposed that inadequate portion of the currently practicing medical profession for all it is worth—from the egotistical attitudes which prohibit diagnosis, to the fraternity that exists between some physicians, (clouding their objectivity through reliance on inaccurate peer influence; covering up the mis-

* Intentionally, to keep the story flowing, only the more remarkable neurologists' visits were documented.

diagnosis by others in their field), to the insurance companies that dictate whether a patient is sick enough for hospitalization—to use today's vernacular, it sucks!

Update

An M.R.I. conducted subsequent to my return home confirmed two additional strokes. I'm currently under the regular care of Dr. Michaels and a competent, compassionate neurologist. In an effort to stifle future strokes, a trial of low-dose chemotherapy was recently prescribed. Unfortunately, it proved ineffective. I've been told the small blood vessel damage deep in my brain is irreparable.

In disbelief, I hear myself admit to Dr. Michaels a thought I hadn't dared consider in the privacy of my own mind, yet. "If I weren't such a strong Catholic—not to mention part of a family who means the world to me—I wouldn't hesitate to contact a physician who advocates doctor-assisted, compassionate suicide." His back to me as he washes his hands at the stainless steel exam room sink, I'm unable to read his reaction to the disconcerting reality I unexpectedly blurted out, other than momentary silence except for the running water. Eddie's sad, lowered eyes and solemn expression, as he speechlessly blends into the chair across from the exam room table are impossible to miss, however.

The unscheduled visit is the result of middle of the night pain so intense, I didn't expect to see morning. Doubled over with severe abdominal cramping so intolerable that the weight of a sheet was more than I could bear, chills surged spasmodically throughout my body. Persistent heartburn felt like a red hot coal lodged in my esophagus, obstinately defying the medications I took to attempt to counteract it. Excruciating head attacks occurred respectively, precipitating other symptoms including nasal and oral intermittent bleeding. Continually suppressing the urge to vomit, every position I tried was equally uncomfortable.

My mind was inundated with thoughts that reflected the fears my condition generated. Was I about to die? Should I have gone to the Emergency Room, even knowing there was nothing they could do? Would it be easier to die there? Instead, as I watched Eddie sleep peacefully beside me, I nervously endured the night—awake and more ill than words could describe.

Exhausted by morning, I called my dad whom I previously promised I'd help pack for his move to another apartment. Though he expected me for 9:00 a.m., knowing he's an early riser, I took advantage of the situation and changed the time to 7:30 a.m., thinking the sooner I was done, the better my chances of getting back in time to see if my doctor could squeeze me in. At the moment, my priority was my dad—I wasn't about to disappoint him.

Working diligently though weak and tired, I tried to use the time as efficiently as possible. I boxed pantry items, wrapped dishes, hung shirts in dry cleaner bags and discarded unwanted items in the dumpster. When he asked me to clean out his dish drainer, I had to steady myself against the counter, grateful he was oblivious from where he was working in the living room. At one point, as I emptied the contents of his medicine chest, I caught a quick glimpse of myself in the bathroom mirror. The fatigued, bloodshot eyes, pasty white complexion and colorless lips of the countenance that stared ominously back at me confirmed that I looked every bit as deathly ill as I felt. Unnerved, I quickly averted my gaze.

My job completed, I arrived home in the afternoon and called Dr. Michaels' office. I was relieved that he was willing to extend his already long day to see me—and even more grateful that the early evening appointment coincided with a time when Eddie would be home to drive me. In the interim, as the previous sleepless night combined with the day's activities caught up with me, my body gave in to the overwhelming fatigue. The essential nap was short-lived, however. Within ten minutes, I awoke to eyes tearing from uncontrollable choking on saliva I neglected to automatically swallow, as people normally do in their sleep.

Dr. Michaels' empathy is undisguised as he verbally acknowledges that I live a horrible physical existence—one for which no effective treatment exists. As though suddenly remembering I'm not the only one clinging to his words, praying for some sign of hope, he faces the husband desperate for an answer and apologetically states, "I don't know what to tell you, Ed"—all the while knowing that admission, honest though it may be, is not what he wants to hear. Scared and dejected, we leave his office fearful of what the next episode will bring.

1997: A Year of Happy Times; A Year of Sad Times

Continued residual symptoms excluded, this year has had a monumental influence on my life. It's been an emotional roller coaster, a ride at times I wanted to last forever—and at others, I wanted to jump off midway, pretending it never happened.

Storey's Graduation

With mortar board cap still in hand, attired in her white satin Graduation gown with powder blue sash, denoting National Honor Society Membership, Storey prepares to leave for the ceremony. Students are required to arrive an hour before guests. At the beep of her ride's horn, I give her a hug, kiss the top of her head and, with pride misting in my eyes admit, "I've been waiting for this moment forever". With a sweet smile and a return hug, she's out the door.

Ironically, when we first adopted her, a television commercial depicting an Asian valedictorian aired. Standing at the podium looking out into the audience at her beaming Caucasian parents, the student concluded her speech with a smile in their direction and a "Thanks mom and dad". At the time, Storey was just an infant—and that scene nothing more than an unspoken dream in the wishful-thinking minds of her parents. But dreams come true and because this one did, my heart is about to burst with pride as our daughter steps up to the podium and delivers an incredible speech, which we hear for the first time, anxiously sitting at the edge of our seats in the front of the auditorium. Momentarily, I'm reminded of the commercial, as she thanks Eddie and I. But, more importantly, I'm reminded of the special and accomplished daughter Storey is, well-deserving of her acceptance into one of the most prestigious and sought after universities in the country, The newspaper account the next day commented that there wasn't a dry eye in the audience following Storey's emotional speech—I know mine weren't!

A Warm Thanksgiving

With a fully assembled dining room table roped upside down on our car's roof rack, its four legs sticking straight up, rigor mortis style, and a metal bed frame positioned lengthwise down the center of the car's interior, we look like we're right off the set of The Beverly Hillbillies. Instead, were headed to Syracuse for Thanksgiving dinner prepared by Stacey and Tim.

I give them a lot of credit. I'm not so sure at ages twenty-one and twenty-five Eddie and I would've volunteered for such a challenging holiday meal, particularly while at the serious dating stage, when it's only natural to be more insecure cooking for the people you hope to be your prospective in-laws. So let the passengers in other dinner-bound cars continue to gawk. Within hours, as Eddie, Storey, my father, Tim, Stacey, Tim's parents, his sister Cathy and I gather around the same table to offer thanks, the stares will long-since-be-forgotten, replaced with warm memories of the first Thanksgiving shared by two families living states apart, brought together through their children's love. With pride, my dad comments, "I never thought the day would come that I'd be going to my granddaughter's for Thanksgiving dinner." The sentiment confuses my emotions, as my lips curve into a smile while my eyes fill.

Opening the door of the hallway leading to the apartment, a whiff of homemade applesauce invades our nasal passages, tantalizing our taste buds, while the unmistakable aroma of the combined scents associated with a traditional Thanksgiving feast pleasantly overpower us. Teasingly, Stacey, who called me several times for advice regarding recipes says, "Oh, Mom, by the way, when should I put the turkey in?". The question, asked an hour before dinnertime, elicits the humor she intends.

By the time Tim's family arrives, within a half hour of us, the well-traveled table is festively set. Per usual, our visit with our new-found friends is comfortable and unpretentious. Together we share a scrumptious turkey dinner, right down to the homemade stuffing. It is a meal that truly does justice to the effort Stacey and Tim obviously expended. Unmistakable pride registers in the eyes of all four parents and "Pa-Pa Red", while Cathy and Storey are slightly in awe, probably amazed that their siblings pulled it off—or possibly pre-occupied with the thought that they might be expected to do the same someday—a scary scenario when you're eighteen. Though subtle, looks of satisfaction pass, deservedly, between Stacey and Tim as they taste the success of their efforts.

As Tim's mom and I work comfortably, side-by-side, restoring the kitchen back to order after dinner, we share our combined approval of the soul mates our children selected. Each of us has come to love the other's child—and enjoy sharing time with their families. And from the looks of things, there will be more opportunities as none of us doubt marriage is in their future.

Watching her interact with Stacey, the love she has for our daughter is obvious. What I don't tell her, because I can't bring myself to say the words that torment my thoughts, is that Stacey may someday need her more than she knows, given my tenuous health status. She's a good mom and I'm confident that, should the need arise, she'll be there for her. There is sadness and relief at the same time, as that reality weighs heavily on my mind.

After coffee and more dessert than we could finish in a week, Stacey and Tim take us to an animated holiday light show in a local park. To Christmas music playing in the background, we drive through an illuminated wonderland of characters throwing balls through basketball hoops, enchanting castles, and gingerbread people doing handstands and flips against the dark night sky.

After such a spectacular display, we're filled with holiday spirit as we head to our motels.

It was with a warm feeling, of special time shared, that we said our good-bye's the next morning. Before leaving, Eddie took Tim's mom aside and expressed sentiments that summarized the way we both feel. "It would be an honor and a pleasure to have Stacey marry Tim and become a member of a family we like so much". We all agreed it was a warm, memorable Thanksgiving—one that I hope becomes a tradition.

Trixie

The cough Trixie developed a few months ago concerns me, particularly with the sudden addition of shortness of breath and the inability to walk a flight of stairs without stopping, midway, to rest. However, when this typically healthy friend finally concedes to seeing a physician, though he, too, questions her cough, it is only in terms of whether she "finds it stressful raising teenagers". Advising her to take some time out for herself, she's sent home with cough syrup. Yet the cough persists.

I can distinctly hear weakness and breathlessness, in her more labored speech, during our out-of-necessity shorter than usual daily calls. Urging her to return to the doctor, she counters, "Why bother? He thinks I'm a hypochondriac." A relatively new patient to him, he doesn't know the Trixie I do—the one who has been employed for thirty years with the same company, working her way up the ladder to a well-respected position. Nor does he know she rarely took a sick day, except when left with absolutely no alternative. And at that, she often worked from bed when absent. She's one of the hardest workers I've ever known, both on the job and off.

No, something's wrong. I can sense it. We're too connected for me to miss the physical changes that have come over her. And I'm worried. Unrelentlessly, I'm all over her case to return to the physician and/or get a second opinion. At the very least, I suggest blood work. By now, with the cough persisting undeterred, the breathlessness increased and the addition of some bruising, she listens more seriously.

Following her early morning appointment, she calls me insisting she feels fine. Because the blood work was done STAT, (the immediacy of which leaves me with unspoken concern), she'll have the results later today. Relieved that she went back, yet fighting an ominous gut feeling, I speak from experience as I try, as nonchalantly as possible, to prepare her. "Trix, don't be surprised if they admit you." "Yeah, right, they don't even believe I'm ill", she retorts. "With my luck, it's probably cancer", she responds lightheartedly, the tone of her voice convincing me she doesn't really think that. Cringing inwardly at the suggestion of such a foreboding pronouncement, our conversation ends.

Hours later, as I'm preparing dinner, I pick up the phone to Trixie's, "Well, you were right!". "Right about what?", I ask, long since having forgotten what she's referring to. "I'm in the hospital", she continues, and then, after a pause, in a scared voice I'm not used to associating with her, she stammers, "with acute leukemia." Shutting my eyes tightly, I don't know what I was expecting, but certainly not this, as my blood runs cold and I'm suddenly lightheaded.

This can't be happening—not to the friend I've had since the age of eight. Not to the friend who told me she could never watch the movie "Beaches" with me, since I've become so ill—particularly the part where Bette Midler tells her dying best friend that she has a very good memory, to which the friend replies something to the affect that she's counting on it. The sad, unspoken request behind that tear-jerking comment is that she'll share those memories with her surviving daughter someday. My first reaction is denial. "They can't know that already!" But somehow, as I hang up the phone and burst into tears, deep down in my heart, I know they do.

Sitting in Trixie's room waiting for her to get back from x-ray, I can hear the sound of her voice joking with the orderlies, alerting me of her imminent return. Her jovial mood and characteristic teasing, the minute she sees me, fail to prepare me for the unexpected and dramatic transformation in her facial color. I have all I can do to camouflage shock as my friend's black and blue, in some spots purplish, bruised-looking face comes into view. But I have to for her sake.

As her uninterrupted chatter continues, her mood seems void of the concern I experience looking at her. The thought occurs to me that she hasn't come to terms with assigning her situation the gravity it deserves—a revelation confirmed by a subtle, passing look of fear I detect in the eyes of her life-long male friend, who re-enters after speaking to the doctor. His arrival is just in time to hear her upbeat report, that she feels fine and her leukemia is the curable type. His perceptiveness prompts him to walk me to the elevator when I leave, detouring me first, the minute we're out of earshot, to a family room down the hall.

Alone with him in the privacy the room affords, I burst into tears—tears that needed to fall, but I somehow concertedly held back until now, for Trixie's benefit. As my rubbery legs collapse, I drop onto the nearest couch. Face buried in hands saturated with sobs generated by the grave physical condition of the friend I love, I feel an arm around my convulsing shoulders. As gently as possible, while at the same time preparing me, he confirms my worst fears, "Her case is far too advanced to respond to treatment. The doctor says she probably won't make it through the week. They're doing everything they can to keep her as comfortable as possible—but we're going to lose her." Sputtering incoherently, I ramble, hearing myself say words I'm thinking but don't consciously share, as I reminisce aloud. Of the verbalized thoughts that can be deciphered, I convey "But she's my very best friend. This can't be happening to her, of all people. She's always been so strong. And we're so close. We talk on the phone everyday. We just went out for breakfast, together, last week. There's nothing I can't tell her. She's like a sister to me—we can count on each other for everything. I can't imagine life without her." Caught up in my own little world of memories, I vaguely hear the "I know darlin", he soothingly repeats in response to my outbursts.

Yet all the comforting in the world doesn't change fate. Though Trixie fights with every ounce of strength, remaining alive far longer than her prognosis dictated, shortly after Thanksgiving I lost the best friend I ever had—or ever will, aside from Eddie. No one could ever fill the void in my life created by her absence. Part of me still doesn't believe she's not here, and that this is just a horrible nightmare. I find myself wanting to pick up the phone and call her as instances we'd normally share, occur. And then I remember—I can't.

Ironically, after having committed her phone number to memory hundreds of calls ago, during the last few months prior to her passing, I had a mental block—requiring me to look it up every time. Coincidence? Or was God trying to prepare me, too?

I never delivered a eulogy before, but somehow, hard as it was, it felt right in this case. I related how we first met in third grade, told of the monumental influence we'd had on each other's lives, and eluded to the fact that there are many, many confidences we shared over the years—all of which will remain undisclosed forever, locked in the privacy of our minds. I assured her children, whom she adopted, that as an adoptive parent, myself, chosen children are wanted children—and that she wanted them so much. They were her world. "Because I loved your mom, it's only natural that I love each of you—and always will", I concluded.

Looking directly into the sobbing eyes of her beautiful daughter, facing me from her seat in the first row, I had all I could do not to burst into tears, halfway through, and run to comfort her. But I had to share these thoughts in their entirety: for her family's sake, for Trixie's, and for mine. I willed my emotions to remain in control, in contrast to the inconsolable state I was in at her wake the night before—at least until I got through it.

A few days previous, I had the eulogy I prepared professionally done in script, on a subtle and peaceful background of the sky, layered in pastel shades of salmon, beige, lavender and blue. Across the bottom, resting horizontally on what appeared to be sand at the ocean's edge, was a single, long stemmed red rose.

It was mounted in a cherry wooden frame, which complimented the serene paper I intentionally selected. When I had it done, it was with the intent of presenting it to her only daughter, on my way back to my pew after reading from it. Looking into her love-generated, tear filled eyes, aching inside as I watch them stream down her face, I thank God I had the foresight to prepare this keepsake. Stepping down from the podium, I walk over to her seat, kiss the top of her head, and hand it to her.

Returning to my pew, having gotten through delivery of one of the most difficult talks I've ever given, I bury my face in hands resting on my lap and cry the tears I've intentionally held back—tears that need to fall. For today I said good-bye to my best friend, whom I love and will miss dearly. At my side is the only other best friend I'll ever have, rubbing my back consolingly. Minutes later, Eddie and I leave the church, hand-in-hand.

Gotcha!

"Hi, Mom, I was wondering if, by chance, you and dad are going to be home on Friday evening", Stacey's voice nonchalantly inquires long-distance. "We can be. Why?", I reply. "Well, it's no big deal but Tim has a meeting at his home office in Connecticut and will be traveling from New York to attend. Since I don't have class that day, I'm planning on going along to keep him company during the ride. We thought if you were going to be around, we'd stop in and visit. Now that I know you are, how about if we spend the night?", she casually suggests. "That sounds wonderful. I miss Trixie so much, your visit will be a welcome lift—as were the beautiful flowers and adorable teddy bear you and Tim sent me when you heard I lost her. And this way you'll get to see them, too." "By the way, Mom, how are you adjusting? Dad E-mailed me that you've been so sad. I wish I could do more." "You already have, Stacey, just by being you. I think this is going to take a long time to accept. I miss her more than you can imagine." "I know how much she meant to you. When I lived home, she's the person I remember calling you most. It must be just awful", she acknowledges empathetically. "It is", I admit honestly, my eyes filling.

Since Stacey's favorite holiday is Christmas, I know it takes a lot for her to say, "Mom, don't worry about decorating the house. With losing Trixie, I'm sure you've got a lot of other things on your mind." Whether she realizes it or not, the timing of her up-and-coming visit is the best therapy in the world for me. Stacey's right, I'm not prepared for the holidays. The house doesn't twinkle like a Christmas shop as it customarily does by early December. I haven't made my traditional variety of cookies, one different batch per day, starting Thanksgiving weekend, (to be frozen in anticipation of the holiday), baking through mid-December. There are no cards displayed and a year's accumulation of dust still coats tapes of my favorite Christmas songs. But I have four days—and a lot of determination!

By the time Stacey and Tim walk in Friday evening, the smell of gingerbread baking permeates the air, in a house illuminated with so many strands of tiny white lights no lamps are needed. Two Christmas trees are fully decorated, one traditionally and one with teddy bears, which I collect. Seasonal candles, Christmas placemats, a hand-painted village, (complete with skating rink), and over a hundred cards are displayed. Holiday music plays in the background, as the look in Stacey's eyes reflect the sentiment painted on the wooden heart, annually hung inside the wreath on our entry door: "All hearts go home for Christmas for love is always there." Deep down, I know this is the house she wanted to come home to—just the way it looks tonight. Her look of appreciation is worth every hour it took to decorate.

Even before taking off her coat, she asks, "Where's dad?" getting her answer as he walks into the kitchen. "How did your meeting go, Tim?", Eddie asks. With a look I can't quite read transforming her face, Stacey hesitates. "Well actually, Tim didn't exactly have a meeting today. We drove all the way from Syracuse, after he got out of work, to show you this", she admits with heightening excitement in her voice as she extends her hand, displaying a beautiful diamond engagement ring.

Mouth open and eyes gaping, I'm in speechless surprise. Through glistening tears, her diamond sparkles beyond its own natural radiance. Throwing my arms around her, I'm stunned and thrilled at the same time. Stunned because as much as they've been dating each other exclusively for the past few years—and I've been expecting it—I erroneously assumed it would coincide with an occasion, such as Christmas Day, her birthday, Valentine's Day or Graduation; Thrilled because Eddie and I have come to love Tim as a son.

With the love of a genuinely happy mother-in-law-to-be, as Eddie hugs Stacey, I embrace Tim, telling him "We couldn't be happier knowing you're about to join our family—as a son". While Tim and Eddie shake hands, I need to sit down, still in a state of shock over an early surprise I've dreamed of since I got to know Tim.

Looking Back

1997 was a year of happy times, a year of sad times. Besides continued illness, there were other losses in addition to Trixie. A first cousin with whom I experienced unforgettable and wonderful childhood memories died prematurely, while an aunt I loved, though she lived a full life, left our family missing her dearly. On the flip side, our daughter Storey was valedictorian, I've been blessed with a beautiful new niece, Alyssa, and Stacey and Tim are engaged. Indisputably, it has been a year of turmoil, characterized by highs and lows.

On Christmas Eve, as our extended family joins us in breaking bread, I do the honors. My voice cracking, I share, "I didn't know how I'd get through this Christmas with the loss of Trixie—and then Alyssa, whom I love dearly, was born. Shortly after, Stacey became engaged to Tim, a person I'm proud to introduce as my son-in-law-to-be. Though nothing will bring Trixie and our other loved ones back, God came through in various ways to help us endure. Merry Christmas, everyone."

Reflections

I reflect often on the impact of the last two and a half years of my life, as a result of that unforgettable light show. When I do, I'm in awe that a person could sustain any semblance of function given the systemic transformation that occurred.

Trapped within the confines of this body, pain rages out of control. With few visible signs on the outside, it remains undetected by others. Yet the invisible monster intensifies by the day, invading every area of my being with its life-threatening presence.

With Central Nervous System damage sustained from that one regrettable incident, I'm no longer the person I once was. An altered internal temperature mechanism leaves me bundled in sweaters and afghans in ninety degree weather as daily I contend with bouts of electric-like chills, one minute on, one minute off. These episodes, which can last for hours at a time, are characterized by a temperature drop of four degrees and associated with doubling over cramps.

I continue to see the world from a blurry perspective and am afraid to go to sleep at night because involuntary jolting in my head awakens me, repeatedly, to thousands of pin-dot lights against a pitch black background. Meanwhile, novocaine-numb appendages leave me desperately trying to shake life back into them.

I've learned to compensate for awakening with suffocating urgency by not allowing myself to fall asleep on my back. Some fears are not that easy to conquer. With each indescribably intense headache, not only do I suppress the strong urge to vomit, but, more importantly, I worry that this will be the one that does me in—and pray that it's not.

Meanwhile, I try to get through the pain one day at a time, hopeful that the near future will bring improved technology and long-awaited relief. In the interim, Eddie and the girls are my most effective incentive to keep fighting. I just pray I have enough fight left.

In writing her essay for college admission, Storey told me that she wanted to write about something that impacted her life significantly. She went on to say, "Everyone has something that influences the person they are" and I thought, how true. Be it color, prejudice, poverty, adoption, isolation, prison—whatever, the experience molds its impact on you indelibly. It controls and shapes the way you respond to certain situations and your future, in general. Twelve years of severe illness, which, for the most part was denied by physicians, (connective-tissue diseases can take a long time to definitively diagnose), drained me in some ways and strengthened me in others.

Undeniably, in the words of one physician, I've been through "Medical Hell". One thing is certain, I will NEVER be the same as a result of this experience. For the most part, the way the majority of physicians I consulted treated me is responsible for the irreparable loss of credibility I now feel toward them. Unfortunately, I fell through the cracks of the medical system—with devastating consequences, both physical and emotional. On the other hand, a degree of fight and determination, laced with assertiveness far superseding what I ever thought capable of possessing, materialized.

In retrospect, writing this book provided a healthy and necessary outlet—one undoubtedly responsible for any sanity still intact. At times, the pen seemed self-propelled, as one idea flowed into another, sharing an intimate part of me I never thought I'd have the courage to publish.

A recent note from Storey...

Mom,

I wanted to let you know what an amazing person I think you are. To battle an illness and still lead a fairly normal life is remarkable in itself, not to mention creating an entire wedding pretty much single-handedly. I know sometimes you must feel underappreciated and, at times in my life, and I'm sure in Stacey's, it is easy to forget to show you how much we care about and admire you.

When I saw the painting entitled "White Companion" on this card, I was incredulous over how accurately it expressed how I feel about you and your support. Then I read about the artist in relation to this painting and I thought it fit even better. Although I am no art expert, I'd like to share my thoughts with you.

Chu Hing-wah, the artist, works with psychologically disturbed patients. He learns from his interactions and has developed a sense of the similarity between all people in terms of their emotions. He tries to capture emotions in his paintings. In this particular one, his daughter posed for the girl. Furthermore, he personifies flowers in his paintings by eliminating certain things like stems and leaves. He uses sparse geometric representations to add a sense of order to the emotionally disturbed...or so it seems to me in this painting of what appears to be a sad, lonely and perhaps unsure girl. The flowers, white and geometric, offer life, stability and a shoulder to lean on. They are comfort and assurance in a world where, sometimes, the girl, the daughter, feels detached and isolated. What I'm trying to say is you are my White Companion — a truly amazing woman — and I love you.

Storey

Appendix

Stroke: An Overview

The American Heart Association, The National Stroke Association and The National Aphasia Association provide comprehensive educational material to the public. The information included in this section was extracted from literature obtained from all three organizations.

What is a Stroke?

A stroke is an attack that occurs in the brain. It results from oxygen and nutrient deprivation caused by an interruption in blood flow to a specific area. When brain cells do not receive these necessary components, carried by the blood, they die. With nerves damaged at the site of the attack, depending upon what function within the body those specific nerves controlled, a victim can experience a variety of limiting, residual symptoms. These include memory loss, incontinence, paralysis, swallowing difficulty, speech problems and visual disturbance, among others. The affects of a stroke can run the gamut from mild to fatal. Though some symptoms are irreversible, with time and rehabilitation, others are not.

How Many Types of Strokes Are There?

Strokes fall into two categories: Ischemic, (is-KEM-ik), or Hemorrhagic, (hem-o-RAYG-ik).

Ischemic Strokes

Ischemic strokes result from narrow or clogged blood vessels, blocking blood flow to the brain. They are the most common, responsible for three out of four strokes. Ischemic strokes are characterized by symptoms developing within minutes or progressing for hours. Often preceded by T.I.A.s, (transient ischemic attacks, defined in greater detail later in the text), they can result in loss of strength to one side of the body, language and speech difficulty and visual or balance irregularities. Most ischemic strokes occur at night or in the early morning. Ischemic strokes fall into three categories: Thrombotic, Embolic and Systemic Hypoperfusion.

Thrombotic Stroke:

Frequency: 60% of all strokes

Characteristics: Caused by a thrombus, (blood clots in an artery, blocking blood flow to part of the brain). Often occurs in an artery damaged from arteriosclerosis.

Embolic Stroke:

Frequency: 20% of all strokes

Characteristics: Caused by an embolus, (wandering clot), developed somewhere else in the body, such as the heart or neck arteries. The bloodstream carries the clot to a vessel leading to the brain, blocking it.

Systemic Hypoperfusion, (low blood flow)

Characteristics: Caused by circulatory failure initiating from the heart. Too little blood reaches the brain due to faulty pumping action. Strokes such as these can occur as a result of a heart attack.

Hemorrhagic Stroke

A Hemorrhagic stroke is not the result of a clot. Instead, it occurs when a blood vessel ruptures near or in the brain. Responsible for about 20% of all strokes, they are more fatal than Ischemic strokes. The symptoms, which come on suddenly, can worsen rapidly at times—to the point of coma. This kind of stroke, characterized by severe headache, nausea and vomiting, tends to target younger victims. Hemorrhagic strokes do not usually exhibit early warning signs. They can occur at any time but are particularly associated with accelerated activity. Hemorrhagic strokes fall into two categories:

Subarachnoid (sub-ah-RAK-noid) hemorrhage

Characterized by: A blood vessel rupturing on the surface of the brain, bleeding in between the brain and the skull. Usually, a ruptured aneurysm, resulting from high blood pressure, is the cause. However, there are other, less common reasons for Subarachnoid hemorrhage, including:

1) AVM rupture, (arteriovenous malformation)
2) Internal injury bleeding
3) Venous or capillary problems

Intracerebral hemorrhage

Characterized by: Bleeding deep into the tissues of the brain, associated with chronic high blood pressure.

Who Gets Strokes?

It is estimated that there are 500,000 strokes occurring annually in The United States. In our country, on the average, someone experiences a stroke every minute. Stroke is the leading cause of serious disability in The United States, accounting for half of all patients hospitalized for acute neurological disease. More males than females suffer strokes, with the incidence for each increasing with age. The fatality rate is higher in Blacks than Whites, with the chart I consulted void of rating other races. However, with improved technology and early intervention, the death rate has declined significantly.

What Are the Warning Signs of Stroke?

- Sudden weakness or numbness of the face, arm and leg on one side of the body.
- Sudden dimness or loss off vision, particularly in one eye.
- Loss of speech, or trouble talking or understanding speech.
- Sudden, severe headaches with no apparent cause.
- Unexplained dizziness, unsteadiness or sudden falls, especially along with any of the previous symptoms.

About 10% of strokes receive preliminary warning signs, the T.I.A.s, (Transient Ischemic Attacks), mentioned previously. The symptoms of these temporary brain attacks mimic an actual stroke, with the exception that they last 24 hours or less. They are caused when a blood clot clogs an artery for a limited time, with part of the brain receiving reduced blood flow. T.I.A.s are a major warning sign of brain attack and not to be ignored. People with histories of T.I.A.s are 10 times more likely to have a stroke than others of the same gender and age.

What Can One Do to Lower Their Risk of Stroke?

- Stop smoking
- Lower blood pressure, if elevated
- Low-fat, low-salt diet
- Take off excess weight
- Regular exercise
- Follow doctors' orders, including adhering to prescribed medications and keeping scheduled appointments.
- Limit alcohol intake

References

Ann Landers. *Reader Insists Marathon Shifts Don't Benefit Doctors.* The Hartford Courant, December 25, 1997.

Ann Landers. *Sleep Deprivation of Medical Residents.* The Hartford Courant, March 10, 1998.

T. Stephen Balch, M. D. *Doctor/Patient Relationship.* Volume III, Lupus Erythematosus, 1982.

Susan Campbell. *Journalist Helps to Spread Word About Fighting Against Breast Cancer.* The Hartford Courant, October 30, 1997.

Dr. Ronald Carr. *The Importance of Patient/Doctor Relations.* Lupus Letter, September, 1986.

Charles Inlander and Ed Weiner. *Take This Book to the Hospital With You.* Pennsylvania, Rodalle Press, 1985.

Gina Kolata. *Doctor/Patient Relationships Take a Turn for the Worse.* New York Times News Service. (Reprinted in The Middletown Press, May 8, 1990.)

Ann C. Roark and Robert Steinbrook. *Polls Take the Pulse.* Los Angeles Times. (Reprinted in The Hartford Courant, May 24, 1990.)

Barbara T. Roessner. *Patients the Victims of Medical Residency Boot Camps.* The Hartford Courant.

Howard S. Shapiro, M.D. *The Physician's Ordeal on Becoming Patient.* (Luncheon address given at Lupus Foundation of America Annual Meeting, 1983.)

Resources

American Lupus Society
American Heart Association
L.E. Support Club
Lupus Foundation of America
Muscular Dystrophy Association
National Aphasia Association
National Lupus Erythematosus
Foundation National Stroke Association
Poison Control Center of Connecticut
Taber's Cyclopedic Medical Dictionary
Selectronic's Wordfinder

About the Author

Eileen Radziunas has been exposed to the medical community for years, both as a professional and as a patient. Prior to her diagnosis of lupus, she worked in a physician's office and later joined a physical therapy group. Her search for a diagnosis led her to well over a hundred doctors, representing a myriad of specialties.

With the publication of her first book, *Lupus: My Search for a Diagnosis*, (Hunter House, Alameda, California), she actively advocated lupus awareness. In addition to running support groups and addressing medical students and physicians at YALE and UCONN, she was interviewed by various radio stations and local newspapers. An active participant in numerous speeches, she attended book/author luncheons, library signings and charitable events. Her first book was selected for inclusion in The World Trade Book Show at The Javitt's Center in N.Y.C. She was awarded a scholarship to The Wesleyan Writers' Conference based on submission of sample chapters from *But Doctor, You're Wrong!*. Her primary incentive in sharing such a personal story is public awareness and, hopefully, medical advancement.